AMBLYOPIA

AMBLYOPIA

Max Schapero, O.D.

CHILTON BOOK COMPANY

Philadelphia / New York / London

1596349

Contents

PART I

Introduction

Visual Acuity

Visual acuity is the capacity to discriminate detail or to distinguish form. It may be experimentally or clinically evaluated in terms of four basic thresholds: minimum detectable, minimum separable (resolvable), minimum perceivable misalignment, and minimum recognizable. Each of the four thresholds is measured by a different type of target construction.

Minimum detectable threshold refers to the smallest test object in the visual field that can be perceived. This threshold is primarily a function of the sensitivity of the retinal receptors to light and to the difference in light intensity in the pattern of light distribution which comprises the retinal image of the object and background, and to the sensitivity of the retinal receptors in detecting this differential in light intensity. Typical target content is a disk, square, or fine thin line on a uniform background. The test can be varied by altering the dimensions of the test object, by altering the luminance differential between object and background (in other words, by altering the contrast), by presenting a dark object on a light background or a light object on a dark background, and, in the latter instance, by altering the light intensity of the object. When the target is a small, light object on a uniformly dark background, the test is a measure of the light threshold and the primary factor is the amount of light or quanta absorbed by retinal receptors, not the angular subtense of the object at a reference point in the eye, as it is for other target configurations.

The minimum detectable threshold may be exceedingly low. Under ideal conditions, a thin dark line whose width subtends an angle of 0.5 second of arc at the eye can be detected if the line is of sufficient length (Hecht and Mintz, 1939). The center of the retinal image of such a dark line has a dip in retinal illumination approximately equivalent to a 1-percent reduction from that of the surrounding retina.

Minimum separable (*resolvable*) is the threshold of the ability to perceive two adjacent and simultaneously observed objects as being separate. The smallest angular separation between neighboring target elements at which the elements can be just resolved is a measure of the threshold or resolving power of the eye.

A primary limiting factor is the amount of diffraction undergone by light from the target as it passes over the edge of the pupillary aperture of the eye. Diffraction spreads the image of a point source of light into a central light disk surrounded by a series of alternate dark and light rings (minima and maxima of light intensity) and thus affects the pattern of light distribution in the retinal image of the target. The amount of diffraction is related to the wavelength composition of light and to the diameter of the pupillary aperture. The smaller the pupillary aperture, the greater the diffraction.

The spread of light caused by diffraction alters the sharp boundary between the light and dark components of the target to a series of light and dark bands, which reduces the steepness of the light gradient in the retinal image. For the neighboring light and dark target elements to be perceived as separate, their retinal images must have a sufficient difference in light intensity to be detected by neighboring retinal receptors. Thus, other important factors influencing the minimum separable threshold are the type, size and separation of the retinal receptors and their sensitivity in detecting and signaling a difference in retinal illumination. Additional factors that affect the pattern of light distribution of the retinal image, and therefore the threshold, are aberrations of the eye's optical system, stray light within the eye, and ametropia.

Test patterns commonly used to determine the minimum separable threshold are parallel dark and light lines of equal width (gratings), checkerboard formations, and pairs of light or dark dots or bars. The test can be varied by altering the size or separation of the components of the test target and by altering the level of illumination. The threshold for two light disks, parallel light lines, and gratings has been found to be approximately 1 minute of arc.

Minimum perceivable misalignment is the threshold of the ability to detect the misalignment or alignment of two discontinuous target segments whose ends are in close proximity. The most frequently used test target consists of two straight lines which, when aligned, lie in the same meridian. The smallest meridional displacement of one target segment, in reference to the other, that can be detected is a measure of the threshold or aligning power of the eye (as, for example, the smallest detectable lateral displacement of one vertical line in respect to another, lower vertical line). Acuity based on measurement of the minimum perceivable misalignment or alignment is termed *vernier visual acuity*.

The spatial discrimination of the relative difference, if any, in the meridional location of the two target segments is based on retinal local sign: that is, on the sensitivity of each retinal receptor or receptor unit in registering a specific visual direction. The subjective identification of small differences in visual direction is also a factor in the threshold of stereopsis (stereoacuity). In stereopsis, however, the task is one of appreciating binocular differences in local signs associated with minute differences between the two eyes in the retinal location of image points of two or more objects at different distances in space (in other words, on the appreciation of retinal disparity).

Under ideal conditions, the threshold of the minimum perceivable misalignment can be as low as 2 seconds of arc (a fraction of the width of the smallest cone cell). The threshold is influenced by the separation and length of the target segments and by contrast. The threshold is lowered by increasing the length of the lines and by increasing contrast, and is raised by increasing the size of the gap between target components (within limits).

Minimum recognizable threshold is the ability to name or identify correctly a form or the orientation of a form. (The minimum recognizable threshold is that usually referred to in the clinical use of the term "visual acuity.") Clinically, the standard resolution threshold (or minimum angle of resolution) is taken to be 1 minute of arc. Threshold measurement is based upon the detection of a break in a form of 1 minute of arc when the total angular subtense of the form at the posterior nodal point of the eye is 5 minutes of arc. If the distance between the posterior nodal point and the retina is taken to be 17.0 mm for a typical human adult eye, an angle of 1 minute of arc corresponds to a linear retinal distance of 4.90 microns (equivalent to two or three cone cells at the focal center).

Snellen letters are the most widely used form targets. Each Snellen letter is so constructed that it can be enclosed in a square five times the thickness of its limbs. The width of the limbs and the separation between them are each one-fifth the size of the letter.

Visual acuity determined with Snellen test type is expressed in the form of a fraction (the Snellen fraction) in which the numerator represents a standard viewing distance (as 20 feet) and the denominator represents the distance at which the breaks and the width of the limbs of the smallest correctly identified Snellen test type subtend an angle of 1 minute of arc at the eye's posterior nodal point. Thus, a Snellen notation of 20/20 indicates a test distance of 20 feet and the ability to correctly identify Snellen test type whose width of limbs and breaks subtend an angle of 1 minute of arc; 20/40 indicates that the width of limbs and breaks in the smallest correctly identified Snellen test type subtend an angle of 1 minute of arc at 40 feet and an angle of 2 minutes of arc at 20 feet (the test distance). Therefore, a minimum recognizable acuity of 20/40 is twice the threshold of 20/20 (that is, the minimum angle of resolution is 2 minutes of arc in 20/40 vision and 1 minute of arc in 20/20 vision).

Landolt C is another frequently used acuity test target. Like the Snellen test type, it is based on a minimum angle of resolution of 1 minute of arc for the break in a letter C which subtends an angle of 5 minutes of arc. The width of the limb of the C and its break in continuity are each one-fifth the diameter of the letter and subtend an angle of 1 minute of arc at a specified distance. The breaks in the Cs are placed in different positions, and the observer identifies the orientation or location of the break (up, down, right, and so on). The correct identification of a break subtending an angle of 1 minute of arc at the eye's posterior nodal point corresponds to 20/20 acuity.

The designation of an acuity score when using Snellen or Landolt test type is usually based on the percentage of correct responses as the threshold is approached. Clinically, the correct percentage required for letters of the same size may vary between 50 and 100 percent, but a criterion of between 70 and 80 percent correct is commonly used.

Routinely, in evaluating visual acuity with Snellen letters, Landolt Cs or other form targets, all factors are held constant except the angular size of the targets. However, the letters of the alphabet used in Snellen test type and the spacing between targets may influence the results. Some letters are more easily identified than others, and a small intertarget spacing relative to target size can make identification more difficult.

Reduction of the Snellen fraction to a decimal (the Snellen decimal) is used on occasion to express the acuity score—for example, 0.20 for 20/100. The decimal, however, does not represent the percentage of vision present, because the Snellen fraction represents a threshold or sensitivity measurement. Thus, 20/100 or 0.20 indicates only a minimum angle of resolution of 5 minutes of arc, not that only 20 percent of vision is present.

To state the percentage of useful vision present, the Snell-Sterling visual efficiency scale was devised, which originally was of special use for industrial or insurance claims. The Snell-Sterling notation designates visual efficiency as a function of corrected visual acuity according to the formula:

$$E = 0.836 \, (1/s - 1) \times 100$$

where s equals the Snellen fraction. In this notation, as the minimum angle of resolution increases in arithmetic progression, visual efficiency decreases in geometric progression; 20/20 acuity is taken as 100 percent visual efficiency. Thus, employing this formula, 20/40 acuity is equivalent to 83.6 percent visual efficiency, 20/100 is equivalent to 49 percent visual efficiency, and 20/200 is equivalent to 20 percent visual efficiency.

Factors Influencing Visual Acuity Thresholds

Several physical, physiological and psychological factors influence visual acuity thresholds. Physical factors pertain to the stimulus conditions and to the optics of the eye; physiological factors pertain to the retinal mosaic, to the neural activity from the retinal receptors to the visual cortex, and to oculomotor control; psychological factors pertain to the observer's behavior, mental ability and perceptual skill.

PHYSICAL FACTORS

Stimulus Variables.   Stimulus variables, in addition to target size and content, include the general level of illumination, wavelength composition, contrast between test targets and background, and exposure or viewing time.

An important effect of the general level of illumination is its influence on the state of adaptation of the eye. If the illumination is at a photopic level and the eye is adapted to it, visual acuity will be better than if illumination is at a mesopic or scotopic level and the eye is adapted to that lower level.

The superior visual acuity at the photopic levels results from the functional characteristics of cone receptor cells as opposed to the functional characteristics of a combination of rod and cone cells or rod cells alone at the mesopic and scotopic levels. For maximum visual acuity to be attained, the general illumination should be the same as that of the test field and the eye should be completely adapted to this level, regardless of whether it is photopic, mesopic or scotopic. Receptor mechanisms function most efficiently under this condition.

Contrast between test target and background is usually held constant in routine acuity testing. Typically, targets are black against a white background and provide almost maximum contrast. However, the sharp differentiation in light intensity at the border between the light and dark target areas is not maintained in the retinal image. Diffraction, optical aberrations, stray light within the eye, and ametropia cause light spread that considerably reduces the steepness of the light gradient in the retinal image. With near maximum contrast in the target, however, the brightness-difference threshold is exceeded and thus is not a significant factor in the acuity test. Visual acuity thresholds can be tested by varying contrast, but visual acuity is at a maximum when contrast is at or near maximum.

In clinical acuity evaluation, exposure to test targets is not limited to momentary time intervals. To influence acuity threshold significantly, exposure time must be limited to 0.1 or 0.2 seconds or less. A reciprocal relation exists, within limits, between brief exposure time and target luminance. Thus, an increase in acuity threshold (reduced acuity) caused by decrease in exposure time may be offset by an increase in light intensity. Contrast and angular size of target are also reciprocally related to exposure time; increase in contrast or angular size can offset a reduction in acuity induced by reduction in exposure time. The primary factors involved in these reciprocal relationships are the amount of usable light (quanta) stimulating the retinal receptors per unit time and the difference in retinal illumination between neighboring components of the retinal image for the region of the retina stimulated and the state of adaptation.

Optics of the Eye. The pattern of light distribution in the retinal image of a target is considerably altered from that of the target as a result of diffraction, aberrations, stray light, transmissive properties, and ametropia. Acuity thresholds are increased by these optical effects because the thresholds are closely related to differences in light distribution between components in the retinal image and to the retinal receptors' sensitivity in detecting and signaling differences.

Light undergoes diffraction in passing over the edge of the pupillary aperture; the smaller the pupillary diameter, the greater the diffraction spread of a point image. If all other factors remain constant, the increase in diffraction spread causes a decrease in image quality or fidelity, which results in a corresponding increase in visual acuity threshold. A small pupil also decreases light transmission and thus retinal illumination. As the pupillary diameter decreases, though, the deleterious effects of the optical aberrations of the eye (particularly spherical and chromatic) decrease and the depth of focus increases. The last two effects improve image quality and tend to offset the adverse effects of diffraction and reduced light transmission. The reverse is true as the pupillary diameter increases: optical aberrations increase, depth of focus decreases, and these adverse effects in image formation are countered by a reduction in diffraction and by an increase in light transmission.

As in other optical systems with finite apertures, diffraction places a limit on the resolving power of the eye. The diffraction limitation can be determined by applying the concept of the Rayleigh criterion: two images can just be resolved when the central maximum in the diffraction pattern of one image falls on the first minimum in the diffraction pattern of the other. Resolving power can therefore be calculated by determining the radius of the central maximum (Airy's disk) according to the following formula:

$$a = \frac{1.22\lambda}{d} \text{ in radians}$$

where a represents resolving power, λ represents wavelength in mm, and d represents diameter of pupil in mm. As an example, for a wavelength of 555 nm and a 2-mm pupil, the resolving power of the eye, as limited by diffraction, is 0.0003385 radians or 1.17 minutes of arc (70 seconds). For the same wavelength of light, the resolving power of an eye with a 4-mm pupil is calculated to be 0.58 minutes of arc (35 seconds). Therefore, in an eye with a 2-mm pupil, two bright points can be resolved when their angular separation is 70 seconds of arc; in an eye with a 4-mm pupil, two bright points can be resolved when their angular separation is 35 seconds of arc.

Experimental measurements of the resolution of the eye as a function of pupillary diameter have shown the resolving power to be slightly better than that predicted on the basis of the Rayleigh criterion.

The effects of diffraction on the resolving power of an aberration-free eye can also be calculated by applying the Fourier theory of wave analysis. In such an analysis, computations are based on a test pattern (as a grating) in which the luminous intensity across the pattern varies in accordance with a sine wave function. The peak and trough in each cycle of the wave correspond to the maximum and minimum light intensities. The frequency of the cycle is a function of the number of maxima or minima per unit distance in the light pattern from the target. The sinusoidal wave pattern is modulated as it passes through the pupil of the eye, the light spread due to diffraction causing a reduction in the wave's amplitude (in other words, a reduction in contrast in the retinal image compared to that of the target). The amount of contrast reduction (expressed by the contrast transfer function of the system) is a function of the pupillary diameter and of the number of cycles per unit angular subtense (frequency) at the eye. The contrast-reducing light spread in the image can be determined by applying Fourier's analysis to the sinusoidal wave pattern and to the alteration it undergoes after being modulated by the eye.

Beside diffraction, several other important factors influence resolution capacity. Light spread in the retinal image, as previously stated, is also caused by optical aberrations, light scattering, and ametropia. Additional limiting factors relate to the retinal mosaic and receptive fields, to the interaction between retinal receptors, and to the sensitivity of the receptors in detecting a difference in retinal illumination (the brightness-difference threshold).

Visual acuity is maximal and constant for pupillary diameters between 2 and 5 mm (Liebowitz, 1952), the typical range in pupil size at photopic levels of illumination. As the pupillary diameter increases from 2 to 5 mm, the effects of diffraction decrease while the effects of aberrations increase so as to counterbalance each other. Diffraction becomes a dominating factor in resolution capacity when the pupil is less than 2 mm in diameter, as is evidenced by a progressive decrease in visual acuity in the pupillary diameter becomes progressively less than 2 mm. Optical aberrations, particularly spherical, dominate visual resolution when the pupillary diameter exceeds 5 mm, as is evidenced by a progressive decrease in visual acuity as the pupillary aperture increases progressively beyond a 5 mm diameter.

PHYSIOLOGICAL FACTORS

The Retina. If the emmetropic human eye were free from diffraction and optical aberrations, the primary factor limiting visual resolution would be the anatomical and functional characteristics of the retina. The basic features of the retina that act to limit resolution are the retinal mosaic, the sensitivity properties of the rod and cone receptor cells, the degree of interaction of receptor cells, and the size of the clusters of receptor cells that subserve a single ganglion cell (in other words, the size of the receptive fields). The efficiency of the receptor mechanism in detecting differentials in luminous intensity in the retinal image varies according to the level of general illumination, to any difference between the level of general illumination and that of the targets background, and to the state of adaptation prior to and during stimulation.

The type of receptor cells, their interspacing and the population density, and the size of the receptive fields vary according to the region of the retina. The central area of the fovea is composed entirely of cone cells. There, the cross-sectional diameter of the cone cells is thinnest, the space between cone cells is smallest, and population density is greatest. Its receptive field size is also the smallest, approaching a one-to-one connection, by way of the bipolars, to the ganglion cells, accomplished through the bipolars. As the retina extends from the center of the fovea, cone cells become individually thicker and more sparse, rod cells begin to intermingle with cone cells, and receptive field size increases. In the peripheral retina, only rod cells are present, and receptive field size increases to a maximum.

Cone cells operate most effectively at photopic levels of illumination and rod cells at scotopic levels. Thus, at photopic illumination levels, visual acuity is dependent on cone mechanisms, while at scotopic levels it is dependent on rod mechanisms.

The level of illumination and the state of retinal adaptation to the level also influences the effective size of receptive fields. As the level of illumination decreases from moderate photopic levels to the minimum photopic level and from the highest scotopic level to the absolute light threshold, the inhibitory action of the cone and rod receptive fields weakens, which in turn permits a greater amount of excitation within the receptive field. A similar reaction occurs with adaptation. The greater the departure of the state of adaptation from that which is optimum for the illumination of the test field, the weaker the inhibitory effects within the receptive field.

The effective size of the excitatory rod receptive fields is therefore smallest when the receptors are fully adapted and exposed to the highest levels of scotopic illumination. Correspondingly, the effective size of excitatory cone receptive fields is smallest when the receptors are completely adapted to higher photopic levels of illumination. However, the inhibitory effect for fully adapted cone receptive fields reaches its maximum degree at moderate photopic levels, and an increase in illumination beyond that results in no further decrease in the effective size of the receptive fields.

The resolution capacity of the retina is related both to its sensitivity in detecting a differential in light stimulation and to the size of the retinal area occupied by the pattern of light distribution at threshold detection of the light differential. That is, the smaller the differences in the pattern of light distribution on the retina which can be detected, the better the potential visual resolution. And the smaller the area within which a differential in light stimulation can be detected, the better the potential visual resolution. The brightness-difference threshold (ΔI) varies markedly according to the level of illumination: it is high at photopic levels and becomes progressively lower as the illumination level decreases to the lower scotopic levels. The lower brightness-difference threshold at the scotopic levels is attributable to the functioning of the more sensitive rod receptors.

A decrease in brightness-difference threshold with a decrease in illumination level, however, does not result in an increase in visual resolution. With the increase in the effective size of the receptive fields caused by increased neural excitation and with the function of rod receptors and their larger receptive fields, a larger retinal distance must be occupied by the dip in the pattern of light distribution for the light and dark areas to be differentiated or resolved. For example, the light and dark lines of an acuity grid must be separated by a progressively greater angular magnitude as the luminous intensity decreases. The greater separation of the grid lines provides a dip in retinal illumination which is of greater depth (relative to the peaks) and occupies a larger retinal area. Thus, as the brightness-difference threshold decreases as a result of reduced illumination, the size of the retinal area within which the differences is detected increases and, as a consequence, visual resolution decreases.

The anatomical and functional characteristics of the retina are reflected by variations in visual resolution, which is at a maximum at the foveal center and becomes progressively lower as stimulation shifts to the peripheral retina. Visual resolution for the region of the retina stimulated is at a maximum when the receptors are fully adapted to the level of illumination of the test field. Visual resolution increases as illumination increases through the scotopic levels and, after leveling off at the point of transition between rod and cone vision, continues to increase until a plateau is reached at higher photopic levels. Thus, the finer the "grain" of the receptor cell layer, the smaller the excitatory area within the receptive field, and the higher the level of illumination of the test field (within limits), the better is the resolution capacity of the retina. Resolution capacity of the retina is therefore at a maximum when illumination is at higher photopic levels and when the target's image stimulates fully adapted cone cells at the foveal center. Under such conditions, small differences in the light distribution in the retinal image can be detected within the smallest retinal area.

It is likely that the resolution capacity of the eye under photopic conditions is limited more by the combined effects of diffraction and optical aberrations than by the resolution capacity of the central retina. Byram (1944), for example, found the resolution capacity of the retina for a grid image to be approximately 21 seconds of arc, compared to a calculated diffraction limit of 70 seconds of arc for a 2-mm pupil and 35 seconds of arc for a 4-mm pupil (wavelength 555 nm). In peripheral stimulation, however, the resolution capacity of the peripheral retina is the primary limiting factor.

Ocular Movements. The human eye is constantly undergoing a series of micromovements characterized by rapid vibratory movements, drifts, and saccades or flicks. The question arises whether the micromovements, by causing the retinal image to stimulate a group of oscillating retinal receptors, serves to enhance visual resolution through a scanning or averaging process, whether the constant motion of the receptor surface acts to hamper visual resolution, or whether the movements are of too small a magnitude to affect resolution at all.

Ratliff (1952) investigated the effects of normal micromovements on visual resolution. Resolution thresholds were determined for a grating test target exposed for 0.075 second, and eye movements were monitored during target exposure. Analysis of the data indicated that the occurrence of drifts or vibratory movements during target exposure tended to impair resolution. Keesey (1960) studied the effects of micro eye movements on resolution and on vernier acuity by comparing threshold measurements made under two conditions— one, the normal condition, in which the micromovements caused the retinal image to stimulate different receptors as the receptor surface oscillated; two, a condition in which the effects of eye movement were counteracted so that, despite eye movement, the retinal image constantly stimulated the same receptors. Essentially the same thresholds were found in each instance, stabilization of the retinal image neither enhancing nor impairing resolution or vernier acuity.

PSYCHOLOGICAL FACTORS

Achieving the potential visual acuity thresholds of which the eye is capable depends on a number of psychological factors. The mental capacity to understand the demands of the test, attention to and concentration on the target, cooperation in steadily fixating, motivation to excel, past perceptual experience, and familiarity with the test situation all serve to improve performance in acuity testing. The more of these requirements the patient meets, the more valid will the test results reflect the acuity potential.

Acuity scores are also influenced by the examiner. His talent in achieving rapport with the patient, his ability to clearly describe the test procedure and its demands, his behavior toward the patient during testing, and his ability to execute the test correctly and without delay all influence patient behavior and responses. The examiner's judgment in selecting an acuity test that conforms to the patient's ability, and his objectivity in obtaining, scoring and evaluating responses also bear importantly on acuity scores.

The factors described in this text as influencing visual acuity thresholds refer only to a normal visual apparatus. A variety of organic and functional disorders can also impair, impede, disrupt or destroy the normal operation of the visual process. As a result, the best attainable corrected visual acuity is less than expected for the age level. It is the purpose of this text to describe the causes of reduced or low visual acuity, exclusive of those attributable to obvious ocular pathology, and to emphasize visual acuity defects that are associated with inadequacies in binocular vision.

CHAPTER 2

The Development of Central Visual Acuity

An understanding of the normal development of visual acuity from birth to maturity is essential before discussing any anomaly of visual acuity. One of the earliest evaluations of acuity at early age levels was that of Chavasse (1939). The *least* acuity present in infants was approximated by the Worth Ivory Ball Test. In it, one of five ivory balls ranging in size from 0.5 to 1.5 inches in diameter is placed on the floor about 6 yards in front of a child. The child is encouraged to retrieve the ball, and his speed and accuracy in moving toward it are used as a means of evaluating his visual acuity.

The minimum acuities expected at different age levels, according to Chavasse, are listed in Table I.

TABLE I *Chavasse's acuity levels*

Age	Acuity	Age	Acuity
4 months	20/2500	2 years	20/40
6 months	20/1000	3 years	20/30
9 months	20/240	4 years	20/25
1 year	20/166	5 years	20/20 or better

Chavasse acuity values for the earliest age levels are obviously approximations based on a gross method of evaluation. Many others have since evaluated visual acuity for young age levels.

Slataper (1950) measured acuity for ages in a series ranging from 2 to 82 years. He examined vision through refractive corrections determined with the aid of a cycloplegic and employed the illiterate E test. His findings for young age levels, as interpreted by Weymouth (1963), are shown in Table II.

TABLE II *Slataper's acuity levels*

Age in Years	Acuity	Age in Years	Acuity
1	20/140 (estimated)	7	20/26+
2	20/48+	8	20/24
3	20/46−	9	20/23+
4	20/40	10	20/22−
5	20/33−	11	20/20−
6	20/27−	12	20/20

According to Slataper, acuity continues to improve slowly until the age of 18, when it reaches its maximum, averaging 20/18. His figures are reasonably similar to Chavasse's but show a slower rate of improvement, an average level of 20/20 not being attained until age 12.

Lancaster's findings (as cited by Abraham, 1951) also agree with those of Chavasse. He found 20/1000 at 6 months, 20/200 at 1 year, 20/50 at 2 years, and 20/20 at 4 years. The writer's experience with age levels 3 to 5 is in closer agreement with the Chavasse tables than Slataper's, 20/20 being frequently found at age 4 and routinely at age 5.

More recently, there has been great interest in the states of development of vision and in the visual apparatus at birth and its rate of improvement with maturation and learning. The method preferred by most investigators to evaluate visual acuity in the newborn is the induction of optokinetic nystagmus. It is a type of ocular nystagmus that results when attempts are made to fixate a series of similar objects rapidly traversing a visual field. The target usually employed consists of a series of black and white parallel lines that are vertically orientated. The lines are of known equal width and are moved across the field of vision at known speeds.

A nystagmoid movement results if (1) the angular subtense of the width of each line, as subtended at the nodal point of the eye, is within the resolving power of the eye, and (2) if the speed of movement of the lines is such that sufficient time is allowed for the subject to identify and fixate a line. The eyes pursue the moving line for a brief interval and then make an abrupt return movement.

Schwarting (1954) utilized a device consisting of a black wire attached to a metronome to elicit a following eye movement in infants and preschool children. A series of wires of different diameters was employed; the smallest wire followed was used as an index to visual acuity. According to Schwarting, there was a high correlation between this method and visual acuity as measured with Snellen test letters in adults. The acuities found are recorded in Table III.

TABLE III *Schwarting's acuity levels*

Age	Acuity
6 months	20/400
1 year	20/200
2 years	20/100
3 years	20/50

Gorman, Cogan and Gellis (1957) attempted to evaluate visual acuity in infants by passing a series of vertical lines before their eyes to produce optokinetic nystagmus. At a 6-inch distance, the lines corresponded to a 20/670 Snellen acuity. They tested 100 infants between the ages of 1½ hours and 5 days; 93 demonstrated nystagmus. Since only one set of lines was used, it is likely that better acuities could have been elicited.

Fantz (1961, 1963) performed a series of visual preference experiments on infants and found that they showed a definite fixation preference for complex form patterns. Their preference was interpreted by Fantz as an indication that form perception is already present at birth and is not dependent upon learning for its inception.

Fantz also performed experiments on infants to evaluate visual acuity. In one experiment (Fantz and Ordy, 1959), two targets were simultaneously presented to the infant, one with black and white stripes and one a solid gray. The width of the finest striped pattern found to be fixated in preference to the gray target was used as a means of estimating visual acuity. In another experiment (Fantz, Ordy and Udelf, 1962), a moving striped field was passed before the infant's eyes to create optokinetic nystagmus (as was done by Gorman, Cogan and Gellis). The results in both experiments showed a minimum separable visual angle of 40 to 60 minutes at less than 1 month of age. In terms of Snellen acuity, that corresponds to 20/800 to 20/1200. By the age of 6 months, a minimum separable visual angle of 5 minutes was found, corresponding to a Snellen acuity of 20/100.

Dayton et al. (1962, 1964) performed similar experiments on infants but added electro-oculography to confirm the existence of optokinetic nystagmus in preference to relying solely on visual observation. In one experiment, a tape containing black and clear stripes was moved across the infant's field of vision, the line widths increasing as the tape progressed. Ten infants less than 1 month old were tested; line widths corresponding to Snellen acuities of 20/160 to 20/250 produced nystagmus in 8 infants while 2 premature infants demonstrated nystagmus with line widths corresponding to 20/800 and 20/1000, in terms of Snellen acuity.

The acuities found for the 2 premature infants correspond closely to those measured by Kiff and Lepard (1966), who found that the majority of 44 premature infants, ages 5 to 83 days, manifested visually observed optokinetic nystagmus for line widths corresponding to 20/820 after reaching the weight of 4 pounds.

In a second experiment on 39 full-term infants, 8 hours to 8 days old, optokinetic nystagmus was created by targets of black and white lines of equal width. Three line widths were used, subtending angles at the eye of 7.5 minutes (20/150), 14.9 minutes (20/290), and 22.3 minutes (20/440). As in the first experiment, the target was moved across the roof of a plastic canopy placed over the infant. Of those tested, 13 had records sufficiently clear to permit an evaluation of visual acuity. Nine demonstrated nystagmus with the narrowest line widths (20/150 acuity) as well as with the wider line targets, and 4 responded only to the 20/440 target. A comparison of acuity findings in these experiments is presented in Figure 1.

While the findings of more recent reports vary, they indicate

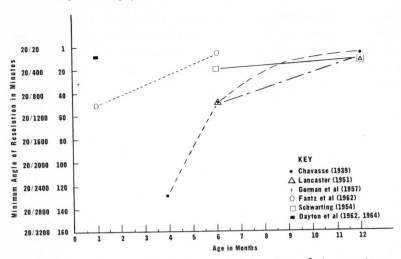

Figure 1. A graphic representation and comparison of six reports on the development of visual acuity from birth to age one. The ordinate is scaled in terms of the minimum angle of resolution in minutes of arc and the Snellen fraction equivalents.

belief that visual acuity is more highly developed at birth and develops more rapidly after birth than had been generally thought.

Other reports confirm the higher state of development of the visual apparatus at birth. Wertheimer (1961) found that a newborn infant demonstrates directional oculomotor response and coordination of the auditory and visual apparatus, turning the eyes in the direction of a click presented next to one ear; Fantz (1961) found that infants under the age of 6 months demonstrate an appreciation for depth by preferring to fixate solid and textured objects rather than smooth flat circles. White, Castle and Held (1964) found that during the first 6 months of life there is rapid sequential development of visually directed reaching. Dayton et al. (1964) found that newborn infants demonstrate both steady and pursuit fixation reflexes and close correspondence of movements of both eyes. Haynes, White and Held (1965) found that accommodative response begins at 2 months of age and operates fairly accurately by 3 months of age.

Although visual acuity, fixation responses, and accommodation improve rapidly after birth, their improvement is dependent upon not only the physical maturation of the visual apparatus but also continued and constant use. For example, should the active fixation reflex of an eye fall into disuse, the skill that might have been present originally can both fail to improve and degenerate to a lower level, or it can even be lost. Similarly, for visual acuity to reach its maximum level, the visual cortex must continue actively to receive, integrate and interpret foveal impulses. If that process does not occur, visual acuity can fail to improve to normal levels and even deteriorate to lower levels.

CHAPTER 3

Peripheral Visual Acuity

In the normal fully developed retina, the most acute vision is derived from the central foveal area. That is so because of the type of cone cells and their great density in this area, their minute receptive fields, and their relatively large cortical representation. As retinal stimulation shifts from the center of the fovea to the peripheral retina, visual acuity becomes progressively lower. Many have evaluated the decline in visual acuity with increasing amounts of eccentricity of retinal stimulation.

Weymouth et al. (1928) studied central visual acuity up to an eccentricity of 85 minutes and, in 3 subjects, found a regular decline in visual acuity in all retinal meridians tested, with the peak at the center of the fovea. A reduction in visual acuity was measured as close as 10.64 minutes from the axis of fixation. The smallest average increase in threshold found for approximately 0.5 degree (31.91 minutes) of eccentricity was 9 seconds of arc, or a change in visual acuity from 20/13 to 20/16. The smallest average increase in threshold for approximately 1 degree (63.82 minutes) of eccentricity was 23.5 seconds of arc, or a change in visual acuity from 20/13 to 20/21. Weymouth et al. suggest that the regular decrease in acuity from zero eccentricity serves as a central sensory gradient that controls the accuracy and stability of fixation.

Jones and Higgins (1947) also found a decrease in visual acuity as stimulation was shifted from the exact center of the fovea. For stimulation of 5 minutes of arc off the fixation axis, acuity was 92 percent of that on axis, and for stimulation of 10 minutes of arc off the fixation axis, it was 75 percent of that present at the fixation axis. Thus, if vision were 20/20 at zero eccentricity, it would have decreased to 20/21.7 at 5 minutes of arc eccentricity and to 20/26.7 at 10 minutes of arc eccentricity.

Adler and Meyer (1935) are in some disagreement with the two reports just mentioned because they found a small plateau for visual acuity in the center of the fovea for an area of 250 microns before detecting a drop in acuity. This corresponds to an angle of approximately 50 minutes of arc.

According to Polyak (1941), the floor of the central foveal pit measures approximately 400 microns across (1 degree 20 minutes or 40 minutes to either side of center), so it is apparent that, for maximum visual acuity to be obtained, fixation must be extremely precise to maintain constant retinal stimulation within this small area.

Others have measured visual acuity for eccentricities extending well into the peripheral retina. In Table IV and in Figure 2 are the findings of Wertheim (1894) as calculated by Weymouth (1958), of Aubert and Förster (1857) as calculated by Murroughs and Walton (1952), of R. Feinberg (1949), and of Weymouth (1955, personal communication).

The findings of Wertheim, Feinberg and Weymouth are in relatively close agreement; if these three reports are used as a basis for approximating normal expected visual acuities for different degrees of retinal eccentricity, the following are obtained: 1 degree: 20/30; 2 degrees: between 20/40 and 20/50; 3 degrees: between 20/50 and

TABLE IV *Variation of visual acuity with eccentricity of retinal stimulation, a comparison of four studies*

WERTHEIM		AUBERT AND FÖRSTER		FEINBERG		WEYMOUTH	
Eccentricity	Visual Acuity	Eccentricity	Visual Acuity	Eccentricity	Visual Acuity	Eccentricity	Visual Acuity
1°	20/33	1°	20/40	1°	20/31	1°	20/30
2°	20/40	2°	20/80	2°	20/42	2°	20/50
		2°52′	20/100				
		3°13′	20/120	3°	20/48		
		3°51′	20/140	4°	20/58		
5°	20/67	4°17′	20/160	5°	20/70	5°	20/95
		7°14′	20/240				
		8°32′	20/320				
10°	20/100	10°13′	20/380			10°	20/160
		14°37′	20/480				
20°	20/180	16°17′	20/900			20°	20/300--
		30°20′	20/2000				

20/60; 4 degrees: between 20/60 and 20/70; 5 degrees: between 20/70 and 20/100; 10 degrees: between 20/100 and 20/160; and 20 degrees: between 20/180 and 20/300.

The information assumes greater clinical significance when it is related to the size of the foveal and macular areas. Using Polyak's figures (1941), the central fovea measures 1,500 microns across (1 micron equals 0.001 mm) and subtends an angle of 5 degrees at the nodal point; the rod-free central area measures 500 microns across and subtends an angle of 1 degree, 40 minutes at the nodal point (50 minutes of arc to either side of exact center). The floor of the foveal pit measures 400 microns across and subtends an angle of 1 degree, 20 minutes at the nodal point (40 minutes of arc to either side of exact center). The small area in the center of the fovea, which contains the thinnest and most uniform cones, measures not more than 100 microns across and subtends an angle of 20 minutes at the nodal point (10 minutes to either side of exact center).

Surrounding the fovea is the parafoveal area, which measures 2,500 microns across and subtends an angle of 8 degrees, 20 minutes at the nodal point. Surrounding this region is the perifoveal area

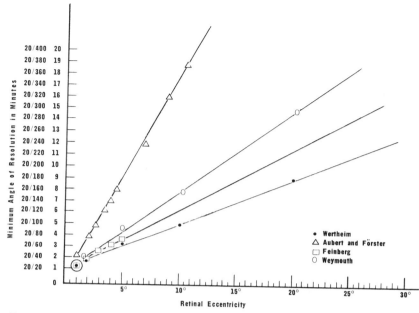

Figure 2. A graphic representation of visual acuity values listed in Table 2 for different degrees of retinal eccentricity. The ordinate is scaled in terms of the minimum angle of resolution in minutes of arc and the Snellen fraction equivalents.

(limit of the macula), which measures 5,500 microns across and subtends an angle of 18 degrees, 20 minutes at the nodal point. The perifovea primarily contains rod cells, with approximately 12 cones per 100 microns, compared to approximately 50 cones per 100 microns at the central fovea.

Should the image of the object of fixation not be exactly centered on the fovea, relating the dimensions of the central area of the retina to acuities found for various amounts of retinal eccentricity would help to determine the best visual acuity. For example, should the image fall at the outer edge of the floor of the foveal pit (40 minutes of arc or 0.2 mm off center), the best expected visual acuity would be approximately 20/25 to 20/30; should the image fall at the edge of the fovea centralis (2.5 degrees or 0.75 mm off center), the best expected visual acuity would be approximately 20/45 to 20/55; should the image fall outside of the fovea centralis but within the parafoveal area (4 degrees or 1.25 mm off center), the best expected visual acuity would be approximately 20/60 to 20/70; should the image fall in the perifoveal area, just within the limits of the macula (9 degrees or 2.50 mm off center), the best expected visual acuity would be approximately 20/100 to 20/150.

Visual acuity decreases at a fairly constant rate as retinal stimulation departs from the exact center of the fovea (Figure 2). The change in acuity with eccentricity of retinal stimulation has been graphically demonstrated by plotting the Snellen decimal as the ordinate against eccentricity of retinal stimulation as the abscissa. Employing this method of presenting the data has led to the erroneous conclusion that the decrease in acuity is at a very rapid rate centrally, changing to a much slower rate peripherally.

For example, if visual acuity is 20/40, the Snellen decimal is 0.5 and is said to represent a 50-percent reduction in visual acuity. That is an incorrect assumption; the Snellen fraction, as we have seen, is designed to be used as a measure of visual acuity in an unreduced form, with the numerator representing the test distance and the denominator representing the distance at which the smallest identified Snellen letter subtends an angle of 5 minutes of arc. By reducing the fraction to a decimal, this meaning is lost. It is obvious that 20/40 vision does not represent a 50-percent reduction in vision, or a 50-percent loss of vision; what it does indicate is that the normal threshold of 1 minute of arc had to be doubled before correct identification was possible.

Weymouth (1958) has convincingly shown that, if visual acuity is represented by threshold values in minutes of arc rather than the decimal of the Snellen fraction and is plotted as a function of eccentricity of retinal stimulation, a straight-line relationship is found. The relationship is present for the central retina, extending to 20 or 30 degrees, beyond which the threshold values increase more rapidly. Weymouth refers to the threshold, when expressed in minutes of arc, as the minimum angle of resolution (MAR). It is readily determined by taking the reciprocal of the Snellen fraction; thus, 20/20 represents an MAR of 1 minute of arc, 20/40 an MAR of 2 minutes of arc, and so on.

By utilizing the MAR instead of the Snellen decimal, Weymouth replotted data from Ludvigh and Wertheim, in addition to his own, and in all three instances the straight-line relationship was found. It indicates that visual acuity decreases in a constant manner for increasing amounts of retinal eccentricity; for an equal incremental change in retinal eccentricity, an equal change in visual acuity occurs. It is not until eccentricity extends to the more peripheral retina that visual acuity drops at an accelerated, not a decelerated, rate.

The above conclusion is opposed to interpretations based on the Snellen decimal rather than on MAR. Visual acuity does not drop at a more rapid rate centrally than it does peripherally. It drops at a constant rate centrally and perhaps at a more rapid rate peripherally.

It is desirable from the clinical standpoint to be aware of off-center and peripheral visual acuities. Such knowledge is especially useful for treating patients who demonstrate below-normal vision that is attributed to continued suppression and/or eccentric fixation. With such knowledge, it is possible to approximate the extent of the central involvement in suppression, or at least the best visual acuity to be expected for a known angle of eccentric or anomalous fixation. But visual acuity for a known, off-center retinal area may be lower than anticipated. That can happen when two or more anomalies coexist, as in the case of eccentric fixation and central suppression. The role that one anomaly, suppression, has played in reducing visual acuity can then be determined.

CHAPTER 4

The Characteristics
of Steady Fixation

Since fixation must be precise to provide maximum visual acuity, the movements characteristic of a normal eye when steadily fixating a stationary target are worth describing: investigations of steady fixation show that a micronystagmoid movement is constantly taking place, together with slow drifts in random directions and periodic rapid flicks or saccades.

Marx and Trendelenberg (1911) conducted one of the best early studies. They fitted an aluminum shell to the eye of one subject and attached a small mirror to the side of the pupillary opening of the shell. Light from the mirror was reflected onto a moving film. They recorded constant eye movements which varied in extent but were usually no greater than 4 to 5½ minutes of arc.

A similar approach was employed by Adler and Fliegelman (1934), but instead of a shell fitted to the eye they placed a mirror directly onto an anesthetized conjunctiva. On the one subject examined, they detected three types of movements: (1) fine vibrating movements occurring at a rate of 50 to 100 per second with an average rotation of 2 minutes 14 seconds of arc, (2) waves occurring 5 or more times per second with an average rotation of from 2½ to 5 minutes of arc, and (3) rapid shifts occurring about once a second with an excursion of from 12.5 to 17.5 seconds of arc. They also noted a tendency for the eye to drift slowly in one direction or another. (It should be noted that Ratliff and Riggs (1950) recomputed Adler and Fliegelman's data and obtained values about one half of those originally computed.)

Ratliff and Riggs (1950) examined five subjects, employing a mirror attached to a firmly fitted scleral contact lens. They found fine vibratory horizontal and vertical movements or tremors occurring at a rate of 30 to 70 cycles per second with a median extent (peak to trough) of 17.5 seconds of arc and rapid shifts or jerks occurring at irregular intervals with an average rotation of 5.6 minutes of arc. They also found slow motions of irregular extent and frequency and slow drifts in random directions, usually not exceeding 5 minutes of arc.

Higgins and Stultz (1953) reported the vibratory movements to occur about 50 times per second, with an average amplitude of 1.2 minutes of arc, while Riggs, in a later work (1952), found them to occur between 30 and 90 times per second with an amplitude of 15 to 20 seconds of arc.

More recently, Hebbard (1957) modified the method of Ratliff and Riggs by placing a mirror on the end of a short plastic rod cemented to a scleral contact lens to eliminate the tear film over the surface of the mirror. He identified three types of movements, similar to those described by Adler and Fliegelman but smaller in amplitude: (1) tremor or micronystagmus of mean frequency of 85 per second with a mean amplitude of 10 to 14 seconds of arc, (2) saccades or flicks occurring every one to two seconds with a mean amplitude of 5 to 6 minutes of arc, and (3) drifts and slow waves.

These small eye movements in steady fixation cause the image to

TABLE V *Summary of data on micro*
eye movements on steady fixation

Source	Micronystagmus	Drifts or Waves	Jerks or Flicks
Adler and Fliegelman (1934)	50 to 100 per sec., 2' 14" of arc average amplitude	periodic, lasting 0.2 sec., ampl. between 2.5' and 5' of arc	every second, 12.5' to 17.5' of arc
Ratliff and Riggs (1950)	60 to 140 per sec., 17.5" of arc median amplitude	irregular extent and frequency	irregular intervals, 5.6' of arc average
Higgins and Stultz (1953)	50 per sec., 1.2' of arc average amplitude		
Riggs (1952)	30 to 90 per sec., 15" to 20" of arc average amplitude		
Hebbard (1957)	85 per sec., 10" to 14" of arc mean amplitude		occurring every 1 to 2 seconds, mean 5' to 6' of arc

oscillate rapidly over a series of retinal receptors in a tiny central area. Since an angle of 1 minute of arc is equal to a 4.90-micron retinal distance, the linear displacement would be minute and stimulation would remain well within the central foveal pit.

In the exact center of the fovea the average cone diameter, according to Polyak (1941), is between 1 and 1.5 microns, equivalent to an angle of 12 to 18 seconds of arc. In this same area the cones are packed more closely, the distance from cone center to center being approximately 2 to 2.5 microns (Jones and Higgins, 1947; Polyak, 1941), equivalent to an angle of 24 to 30 seconds of arc. A micronystagmoid movement as large as 60 seconds of arc would thus move a retinal image point over only a few cone cells.

One interpretation of the vibratory movements, saccades and drifts is that they are the consequence of normal physiological tonus of the extraocular muscles; another interpretation is that micro eye movements are functional and serve to enhance vision and fixation. One reason for the second conclusion is that vernier acuity and stereoscopic acuity may be as low as 2 seconds of arc, one sixth the angle subtended by the smallest estimate of a single central cone cell. It is thus hypothesized that the micro tremors serve as a scanning mechanism to enhance visual resolution, alignment and depth judgments.

If micro eye movements are neutralized and the same retinal receptors are constantly stimulated by the same image content, the vision of the image will fade and be lost. Another function attributed to the vibratory movements, therefore, is that they serve to prevent such a disappearance of images by constantly shifting stimulation to different receptors.

A third use attributed to the micro eye movements is that they act as a feedback mechanism which operates to assist the eye to track and fixate a moving target.

Should fixation not be precisely controlled and should the normal movements associated with steady fixation become grossly exaggerated, visual acuity will be adversely affected. Nystagmus is an example, but less obvious conditions associated with anomalies in binocular vision also affect steady fixation, as we shall see.

PART II

*The Characteristics
of Amblyopia*

CHAPTER 5

Types of Amblyopia

1596349

With but few exceptions, etiological factors of reduced or low corrected visual acuity can be divided into two broad categories, those which are and those which are not attributable to obvious structural or pathological anomalies of the eye. If there are obvious structural or pathological ocular anomalies—in other words, if the cause is observable—the impaired central vision is usually referred to as *low vision, subnormal vision, blindness* or, less frequently, *amaurosis.* Included among such pathological conditions would be corneal scarring, corneal dystrophy, cataracts, keratoconus, aqueous or vitreous opacities, retinopathies, choroidopathies, uveitis, optic atrophy, optic neuritis, papilledema, and colobomata of ocular structures.

If the cause of reduced or low corrected visual acuity is not attributable to obvious structural or pathological ocular anomalies—if it is not observable—the condition is usually called *amblyopia.* Amblyopia may then be defined as low or reduced central vision not correctable by refractive means and not attributable to obvious structural or pathological anomalies of the eye.

The level of vision which constitutes amblyopia may be set by one of two criteria. One criterion relates the vision of one eye to that of the other. If the visual acuity of one eye is less than that of the other, the eye with the lower acuity is considered amblyopic. Using this criterion, an eye with 20/20 may be deemed amblyopic if the fellow eye has 20/15 acuity.

The other criterion, which is more commonly used, relates the maximum attainable visual acuity to that expected for the age level; for example, 20/20 in the fully developed normal eye. If the best visual acuity is significantly less than 20/20, or that expected for the age level, the eye is considered amblyopic. Included in this criterion is bilateral amblyopia, in which visual acuity, though possibly equal, is low in both eyes.

The level of visual acuity constituting a clinically significant departure from the 20/20 expected in a normal fully developed eye varies with the authority. According to Feldman and Taylor (1942), it is less than 20/50; according to Burian (1953), McCulloch (1950) and Costenbader, Bair and McPhail (1948), it is 20/40 or less; according to Schapero (1961), it is 20/30 or less; according to Bourquin (1953), it is 20/25 or less; according to Bangerter (1953), it is 20/25 or less, or less than is indicated by the eye's state of health; and according to Ramsay (1950), it is less than 20/20.

There are essentially two kinds of amblyopia: *functional amblyopia,* in which impairment of the visual pathway is of functional origin, and *organic amblyopia,* in which the impairment is of organic origin (due to nonobservable histopathology). Although the primary emphasis of this text is on functional amblyopia, both types must be considered.

Organic Amblyopia

In organic amblyopia, components of the visual pathway may fail to develop normally because of inherited structural defects, or the functioning of a normal visual pathway may be impaired because of metabolic or toxic disturbances. Depending upon the cause, organic amblyopia is termed nutritional amblyopia, toxic amblyopia or congenital amblyopia.

NUTRITIONAL AMBLYOPIA

Nutritional amblyopia (deficiency amblyopia) refers to loss or impairment of central vision due to dietary insufficiencies or malnutrition, more specifically a lack of the B vitamins, especially thiamine (B_1), riboflavin (B_2), pyridoxine (B_6) and cyanocobalmine (B_{12}) (Dreyfus, 1965). The visual loss is gradual, usually developing over a period of days, weeks or even months. The visual fields typically show a bilateral and roughly symmetrical central, paracentral or centrocecal scotoma, larger for red than for white. Peripheral vision is intact. The fundus remains normal except for a possible temporal pallor of the optic disk. If treatment with B vitamins and adequate nutrition is instituted early, prognosis for the recovery of vision is good.

Ethyl alcohol amblyopia, which at one time was considered a result of toxic effects from prolonged consumption of large quantities of ethyl alcohol, is now considered by practically all authorities to be caused by nutritional deficiencies and to be no different from the nutritional amblyopia found among undernourished nonalcoholics. The alcoholic commonly has poor eating habits, shows signs of malnutrition and will show an improvement in vision with vitamin B therapy even though he may continue to drink.

Postmortem histological studies of the visual pathways of alcoholics who demonstrated amblyopia prior to death have shown a destruction of the medullated nerve fibers of the optic nerve, chiasm and optic tracts corresponding in location to the papillomacular bundle, a thickening and a proliferation of connective tissue in the same areas replacing the medullated nerve fibers, and in some cases a degeneration of the ganglion cells of the retina in the area of the macula.

Victor and Dreyfus (1965) believe that the primary pathological changes occur in the retrobulbar portions of the medullated nerve fibers and that the retina is affected secondarily, which would account for the fact that some investigators have found degenerative changes in the ganglion cells of the retina while others have not. Victor and Dreyfus theorize that the earliest lesions are small bilateral and symmetrical areas of demyelinization, restricted to the papillomacular bundle, which eventually spread centrifugally beyond the confines of the papillomacular bundle. In a histological study on one case reported in 1965, they found symmetrical and extensive destruction of myelinated fibers of the temporal and ventral portions of the optic nerves. Destruction in the distal portion of the nerve, in the region corresponding to the papillomacular bundle but more proximal, was more extensive, involving two thirds of the myelinated fibers.

In an attempt to determine the specific vitamin deficiency involved in nutritional amblyopia, Dreyfus (1965) performed whole blood transketolase studies on two untreated alcoholic patients who had amblyopia. His test reflects the state of thiamine nutrition. The results showed a deficiency of thiamine in both instances.

Added evidence that the responsible nutrient may be thiamine is presented in the study by Carroll (1944), who obtained improvement in vision in amblyopic alcoholics by treating them with thiamine alone. His findings are in keeping with recent evidence that the transketolase activity is greatest in the medullated parts of the nervous system.

Tobacco amblyopia (loss or impairment of vision associated with excessive and prolonged use of tobacco) was also once considered toxogenic. Many authorities now consider this type of amblyopia to fall into the same category as ethyl alcohol amblyopia; that is, to have a nutritional rather than a toxic basis. Others feel that malnutrition, although it may be involved, is not the primary cause, but that the amblyopia is due to some deleterious effect directly attributable to the constant use of tobacco.

Although tobacco amblyopia is sometimes called *nicotine amblyopia,* there is no substantial evidence that it is directly related to the intake of nicotine (Silvette, Haag and Larson, 1960). Some believe it is related to poor health (not necessarily caused by malnutrition) or to vitamin B deficiencies (B_1, B_2, B_6, B_{12}) which may result in a greater sensitivity to the effects of tobacco. In his study of nutritional amblyopia among prisoners of war in Russia, Obal (1951) states that tobacco amblyopia was often eliminated by stopping smoking (usually a pipe).

If tobacco does indeed contain toxic substances which affect vision, the responsible agents have yet to be determined. According to Heaton (1962), the possible toxic substances in tobacco are nicotine, carbon monoxide, pyridine derivatives, arsenic, lead and cyanide. Of these, Heaton believes that cyanide may be the toxic agent. Chronic cyanide poisoning has been found to cause symmetrical demyelinization of the optic tracts which could affect the centrocecal fibers. Normally, cyanide is detoxicated by hydroxocobalmine and hepatic rhondase into thiocyanate.

Heaton states that the secretion of thiocyanate in the urine of smokers rises 6 to 20 mg, which corresponds to the amount of cyanide in tobacco smoke. If a vitamin B_{12} deficiency is present (and such a deficiency has been previously reported in cases of tobacco amblyopia), the cyanide will not be detoxicated, resulting in a rise in the cyanide level, and chronic cyanide poisoning may occur. Heaton believes that a similar effect may be found in those who have diets weak in animal protein. A B_{12} deficiency is likely to be present and the consumption of cyanide in a diet consisting of no meat is likely to be higher than normal.

Rucker (1954, 1960) and Harrington (1956, 1962) believe that tobacco amblyopia is a distinct type of amblyopia, distinguishable from alcohol or nutritional amblyopia. They state that it occurs most frequently in pipe smokers and cigar smokers, less frequently in users of chewing tobacco or snuff, and rarely if ever in cigarette smokers. In chewers and in pipe and cigar smokers, some tobacco residue is swallowed, and some have suggested that this may have some relationship to the cause of the amblyopia (Silvette et al.; 1960).

Tobacco amblyopia typically occurs in males between the ages of 40 and 60 who have a history of long and constant exposure to tobacco. It is characterized by bilateral juxtacecal or cecocentral scotomata which may be more advanced in one eye than the other, the red field being affected earlier than the white. The fundus appears normal. Prognosis is good if the use of tobacco is discontinued, if the disease is not of long standing and if the patient is otherwise in good health. The B vitamins are used in the treatment of this condition.

According to Harrington (1962), the field defect in tobacco amblyopia may be differentiated from the field defect in alcohol or nutritional amblyopia. In tobacco amblyopia, the defect is said to start between the blind spot and the fovea and to extend nasally and temporally to eventually encompass these areas. The scotoma has vaguely defined limits and contains an area of greater density in the juxtacecal location. Since, according to Harrington, the scotoma does not involve the central area in the early stages, it may go unnoticed for some time.

In contradistinction to this picture, Harrington describes the bilateral scotomata occurring in alcohol amblyopia as initially affecting the central area, with an area of greatest density at the fovea and with sharply defined borders. The scotoma is said to extend toward the blind spot with the progression of the disease. Since it affects the central area during onset, this condition is noticed in the early stages. The alcoholic patient may also be a heavy smoker, but his smoking usually involves cigarettes.

If the field defects in these two conditions differ, good evidence is present that they do not have the same etiology. Harrington's findings, however, are disputed by many authorities (Victor, 1963; Adler, 1957; F. B. Walsh, 1957; Duke-Elder, 1941), who claim that there is no consistent difference between field defects and that central, centrocecal or juxtacecal scotomata can occur in either case. Victor (1963) and Victor and Dreyfus (1965) state that pure cases of tobacco and alcohol amblyopia have degeneration of the optic nerve fibers, that there is no fundamental clinical or pathological distinction between the two, and that both have a nutritional basis and respond to vitamin B therapy.

The report of Carroll (1944) is frequently cited to support this contention. Among the 25 amblyopic patients treated by Carroll were those who used tobacco excessively as well as alcohol. Whether the amblyopia was attributed to alcohol or tobacco, or both, all patients showed improvement in vision with dietary supervision or with vitamin B injections or supplements, even though they were permitted to continue to drink and smoke.

Since according to Harrington the primary distinction between tobacco and alcohol amblyopia, in addition to the case history, is the field defect in the early stages, it is understandable that his conclusions would be challenged. In later stages in both conditions, a cecocentral scotoma is present, and field plotting may not have explored the scotoma for areas of greater density.

Because it is agreed that the papillomacular bundle is eventually involved in both instances and because histological studies were performed on advanced cases, the histopathology observed would be similar. Further, many patients in whom both tobacco and alcohol were implicated (tobacco-alcohol amblyopia) were cigarette smokers, a use of tobacco not considered by Rucker and Harrington to cause amblyopia.

TOXIC AMBLYOPIA

Toxic amblyopia is another type of amblyopia that has an organic etiology. It may be defined as amblyopia caused by exogenous poisons, such as methyl alcohol, quinine or lead, or by endogenous poisons, such as focal infections (for example, dental amblyopia).

Both ethyl alcohol and tobacco may produce toxic amblyopia, but the picture is quite different from that described for ethyl alcohol or tobacco amblyopia. Harrington (1962) states that a toxic amblyopia may result from drinking impure ethyl alcohol or whiskey or gin of poor quality and that, in such instances, there is a sudden and marked loss of central vision with large, dense, central scotomata. It is the same type of scotomata found in cases of methyl alcohol poisoning. Victor (1963) states that when tobacco does produce toxic amblyopia, it is characterized by an abrupt onset, rather than a gradual one, and that blindness is often complete.

The field loss in toxic amblyopia may be central or peripheral, depending upon the poisonous agent. Central field defects are produced by such toxins as methyl alcohol, lead, digitalis and ergot, while peripheral field defects are produced by quinine, arsenic and salicylates.

CONGENITAL AMBLYOPIA

Congenital amblyopia, a third type of organic amblyopia, refers to reduced or low vision attributed to congenital or hereditary anomalies in the visual receptors or visual pathways. The visual mechanism fails to develop normally, so visual acuity never reaches a normal level. The condition is more commonly bilateral, but not necessarily so, and it may or may not be accompanied by other congenital or hereditary anomalies. Visual acuity, when maximally developed, usually ranges between 20/30 and 20/200 but more typically is between 20/40 and 20/60.

Examples of other anomalies which may coexist with congenital amblyopia are high refractive errors in both eyes, nystagmus, albinism, color vision defects and motor defects (such as cerebral palsy).

The coexistence of these defects assists greatly in arriving at a diagnosis of congenital amblyopia. Frequently, however, the patient appears normal in all other respects. The problem of diagnosis is then considerably more difficult, particularly if the reduced vision is unilateral rather than bilateral and if there are accompanying visual conditions, such as strabismus and anisometropia, which may indicate a functional etiology.

One condition accompanying monocular amblyopia which offers evidence of congenital etiology is the refractive state of very high anisometropia (as plano in one eye and −12.00 diopters in the other eye). This is especially so when the corrected vision in the eye with the higher refractive error is 20/200 or worse and when there are facial asymmetries and differences in the amount of protrusion of the eyeballs.

A monocular reduction in vision is common in cases of significant anisometropia, but a reduction in vision of less than 20/200 is rare and in itself is an indication of congenital amblyopia. Functional causes of reduced vision affect only the central area, and visual acuity is thus 20/200 or better.

If uncertainty exists concerning whether the amblyopia is congenital or functional after testing has been completed, a training program may be instituted in an attempt to improve vision. Congenital amblyopia is indicated if training is completely unproductive even though carried out correctly for an extended period of time.

A type of amblyopia which may be classified under the congenital category is *receptor amblyopia*. This condition was first described by Enoch (1957, 1959), who investigated the Stiles-Crawford effect No. 1 on a total of six amblyopic eyes. The Stiles-Crawford effect No. 1 refers to the greater stimulus effectiveness (brightness) of a pencil of light ray passing through the center of the pupil compared to a pencil of light passing through an eccentric part of the pupil and stimulating the same retinal point. Five of the six amblyopic eyes examined by Enoch showed an abnormal Stiles-Crawford effect No. 1 (a displaced maximum and/or flattened curves), while the normal eyes showed a normal effect.

Enoch suggests that the abnormal Stiles-Crawford effect No. 1 found in the amblyopic eyes may be due to a simple tilt of the foveal receptors, to a general malorientation of the receptors, to reduced light sensitivity independent of orientation, to a disturbance in the orientation of the internal structures of the receptor cells, or to a disturbance of the photopigment molecules. If his hypothesis is true, reduced vision is caused by an anatomic anomaly and would not improve with treatment. Conversely, if vision does improve with treatment, either the anatomic integrity and orientation of the cone cells is normal or superimposed upon this anatomic anomaly is a functional anomaly which causes an even greater reduction in vision.

Some later evidence casts doubt on the Enoch concept of receptor amblyopia. Campbell and Gregory (1960) investigated the decrease in acuity that occurs when a test target is viewed through a decentered artificial pupil. They found that the acuity loss is primarily the result of optical aberrations of a higher order and that only a small amount of the acuity loss may be attributable to directional acuity of the retinal receptors. Green (1967) has shown that acuity loss due to oblique incidence of light rays, except for that caused by brightness loss, is not a result of directional acuity of the retinal receptors but is caused by optical aberrations of the dioptric system of the eye. These two reports indicate that a defect in the orientation of the retinal receptors, if it did occur, would result in a relatively small acuity loss, the loss being due to a decrease in effective brightness and not to a directional acuity effect.

It is possible that the abnormal Stiles-Crawford effect found by Enoch is a manifestation of undetected eccentric fixation. Marshall and Flom (1968) point out that retinal stimulation of nonfoveal areas can cause a displacement of the maximum of the Stiles-Crawford curve. They measured the Stiles-Crawford effect No. 1 on four amblyopic subjects and found a shift in the peak of the curve away from the pupillary center only when the amblyopic eyes demonstrated eccentric fixation. The shift of the peak was in relation to the magnitude and direction of the angle of eccentric fixation.

Functional Amblyopia

It is presumed in functional amblyopia that the visual pathway is intact and normal at birth but fails to develop or operate normally due to an abnormality in its stimulation or use. Depending upon the cause, vision may develop partially and remain static thereafter, may develop partially and regress, or may develop normally and fully and then regress.

With proper treatment, patients can usually fully recover from functional regressions in vision. Success is more limited when development of vision is lacking, but increased or full development of vision may be attained with corrective measures, depending upon the age of onset and the duration of the inciting condition.

Functional amblyopia, classified according to the type of abnormality involved in the use or stimulation of the visual pathway, occurs in four forms: hysterical amblyopia, light deprivation amblyopia, isoametropic amblyopia and amblyopia ex anopsia.

HYSTERICAL AMBLYOPIA

Hysterical amblyopia (also called psychic amblyopia) may be defined as loss of vision due to a psychogenic cause. In addition to valuable clues from the case history, important diagnostic information may be obtained from examination of the visual fields, which are typically tubular. There is usually a bilateral and symmetrical contraction, and the fields remain of constant size regardless of the test distance.

Other possible variations in the visual fields are spiral (fatigue) fields or star-shaped fields (Harrington, 1956). The spiral visual field is considered an exhaustion reaction. As the field plotting progresses, the limits of the field become continuously smaller. A similar exhaustion phenomenon was found by Krill (1967) in the dark-adapted, peripheral, absolute light threshold. With repeated testing and prolonged dark adaptation, an upward shift in the threshold occurred.

The onset of the reduced vision may be abrupt or gradual (Yasuna, 1963) and, despite the tubular fields and the reduced central vision, the patient appears relatively calm and undisturbed and he demonstrates no problem in maneuvering in space (Wekstein 1949; Harrington, 1956). Unlike one having organically caused low vision or restriction of the visual fields, there is characteristically no complaint of the inability to read or of bumping into objects. Successful psychotherapy may result in restoration of normal central vision and normal fields.

A distinctive type of hysterical amblyopia, or possibly feigned reduced vision, is found among juveniles. Several signs and symptoms typify this condition (Yasuna, 1963; Hirsch, 1965; Meyer, 1966):

1. The patient is a child, typically female, between the ages of 8 and 14.

2. The complaint is a routine one of blurred distance vision which frequently was first detected by an acuity check at school.

3. There has been no history of visual problems or of wearing corrective spectacles.

4. A bilateral and usually equal reduction in visual acuity exists which typically ranges between 20/70 and 20/200.

5. Each acuity target is identified only after prolonged and apparently intense observation, and then with doubt.

6. Findings on external examination, ophthalmoscopy, slit lamp biomicroscopy and ophthalmometry are negative.

7. A minor and approximately equal refractive error (usually a small amount of hypermetropia) exists which is not in accordance with the visual reduction and which does not improve vision.

8. There are no significant muscular imbalances or fusional convergence weaknesses.

9. Cooperation during the testing procedure is good to excellent.

10. Eventual attainment of 20/20 vision with no correction in the phoropter (though the patient is led to believe there is) after proper encouragement.

11. Visual fields may be constricted or tubular or the results of the field test may be inconclusive because of variability in patient responses.

12. There is a history of poor school achievement or an emotional problem related to the school or home environment. A background of social deprivation has also been reported by Hirsch (1965).

The routine nature of the original complaint of blurred vision and referral by the school leads the refractionist to believe that it is probably a simple case in need of a refractive correction, most likely for myopia. The first clue is revealed by the patient's apparent inability to read 20/40 or 20/50 test type and his painfully slow and deliberate (though correct) identification of even larger test types in the 20/200 to 20/100 range. In view of the apparent difficulty in identifying the larger acuity targets, the examiner is likely to conclude that the child will be unable to read the smaller targets and may end the testing before reverting to them.

Suspicions are further aroused when static retinoscopy reveals an insignificant refractive error. The suspicions are confirmed when the subjective examination also reveals a minor refractive error which apparently has no effect on the reduced vision.

At this point, the examiner should suspect the possibility of juvenile hysterical amblyopia, or feigned reduced vision, and alter his examination accordingly. If the child is given the impression by the examiner that he has now put a lens in the phoropter which will make him see better and that the examiner expects him to see better, the child will begin to read smaller test type if abruptly asked to do so. Identification will still be laborious, but by continuing with smaller test type and offering praise and encouragement with each accomplishment 20/20 vision will often be attained even though the phoropter has been entirely cleared of lenses. If now urged to read the same size letters faster, the child will usually comply. The final result will then be essentially normal vision without correction.

The case history may reveal a reading problem or difficulty with schoolwork in general, a sibling or close friend who recently obtained spectacles, problems in learning to play a musical instrument, or a behavior problem at school or at home. The apparently reduced vision in many instances appears to be an attempt by the child to provide an excuse for his poor performance.

There is some question whether the child is consciously feigning poor vision or actually believes he cannot see the letters. No doubt both may occur, but in either instance a psychological problem is present.

The demonstration of difficulty in interpreting acuity targets is frequency of short duration. If the minor refractive correction is prescribed and worn for a short time, a recheck will usually reveal normal acuity with or without the correction. The patient will read the letters quickly and easily and may even be eager to show the examiner how well he can now see.

LIGHT DEPRIVATION AMBLYOPIA

This type of functional amblyopia is attributed to the nonuse of the visual pathway because of a gross insufficiency in the light stimulation of the eye during the first few years of life. Causes of such light deprivation are congenital cataracts, congenital ptosis, traumatic cataracts and extensive corneal opacification.

This form of amblyopia was formerly considered to be caused solely by cortical nonuse, but recent information has indicated that normal development of the visual pathway is also dependent upon or related to light stimulation of the retinal receptors and the consequent use and reinforcement of the synaptic relays.

Experiments on animals have shown that, should the visual pathway be continuously and grossly deprived of light stimulation beginning at or near birth, cells in an originally normal and intact visual pathway develop serious and permanent abnormalities.* Cells in the lateral geniculate body fed by the deprived eye not only fail to mature but appear to degenerate or atrophy. Cells in the visual cortex fail to fire upon stimulation of the deprived eye. The resulting visual loss appears permanent and irreversible.

That a similar reaction occurs in humans is born out by the commonly experienced failure to obtain an improvement in acuity in congenital cataracts after surgery is performed. Even if surgery is successful and the fundus appears normal, the low acuity manifested after surgery typically fails to improve despite adaptation to the refractive correction and extensive visual training. The same irreversible visual loss is found in light deprivation due to traumatic cataract (Juler, 1921), congenital ptosis (von Noorden, 1967) and corneal opacification (von Noorden and Maumenee, 1968).

It is unlike other functional vision disorders in which light stimulation is normal but in which neural inhibitions occur, as in strabismic amblyopia and anisometropic amblyopia. In the latter conditions, visual loss is usually not so severe and vision is usually partially or entirely recoverable. Thus a gross deficiency in light stimulation appears to be a significant factor in contributing to the visual defect and to its permanence.

The earlier in life gross light deprivation begins and the longer it continues to exist, the more profound the effect on the visual pathway. Therefore, surgery for congenital or traumatic cataract or for congenital ptosis should be performed at the earliest opportunity.

ISOAMETROPIC AMBLYOPIA

Isoametropic amblyopia occurs bilaterally and in association with relatively high but approximately equal uncorrected refractive errors

---

* See Chapter 7.

which have been present since early life. It is one of the two types of *refractive* or *ametropic amblyopia*, the other being *anisometropic amblyopia*. Typically, isoametropic amblyopes demonstrate a corrected visual acuity of between 20/30 and 20/60 in each eye on initial exposure to refractive correction. A check of their acuity, after full adaptation to the lens effects, often reveals a significant improvement in acuity which may reach normal 20/20 (Abraham, 1964; von Noorden, 1967). The lower corrected acuity found initially may be attributed in part to unfamiliarity with the lens effects and to the failure to appreciate and interpret fully the improved focus of the retinal image.

The higher the refractive error, however, especially the spherical components, the less likely will normal vision eventually be achieved, probably because of the presence of a developmental anomaly (Duke-Elder, 1963). The portion of the visual reduction which is permanent may be considered an organic or a congenital amblyopia.

AMBLYOPIA EX ANOPSIA

The most frequent cause of functional impairment of vision is the condition of amblyopia ex anopsia, also called suppression amblyopia, obligatory amblyopia, facultative amblyopia and disuse amblyopia. In this condition, the reduced or retarded central vision is attributed to a relatively long-standing suppression, inhibiton, disuse or nonuse of the central impulses from one eye. It is usually associated with unilateral strabismus of early onset (strabismic amblyopia) or uncorrected anisometropia (anisometropic amblyopia) and is also a possible factor in light deprivation amblyopia. Depending upon age at onset and duration, vision may be entirely or partially recoverable through therapeutic means.

In amblyopia ex anopsia, impulses arriving at the visual cortex from the fovea of one eye provide information which is either inferior to or in conflict with the information provided to the same cells by fovea of the other eye. The visual cortex appears to react to this type of bilateral input by responding only to the desirable impulses, the undesirable impulses being inhibited or suppressed.

Frequently, the amblyopic eye fixates with a retinal site other than the foveal center. Such a fixation response would account in part for the low visual acuity present because visual acuity normally decreases in proportion to the increase in eccentricity of retinal stimulation. The visual acuity expected for the retinal area used indicates the portion of the low vison attributable to off-center stimulation.

In some instances, amblyopia ex anopsia may coexist with an organic involvement. The term *relative amblyopia* is given to a condition in which there is a loss of vision not entirely attributable to ocular pathology but partially due to a functional involvement.

Strabismic Amblyopia. The stimulus for the suppression which leads to amblyopia ex anopsia in strabismus is related to the conflicting information fed to the visual cortex by the two eyes. To understand the cause of this conflict in information, it is necessary to be familiar with the concepts of corresponding points, disparate points (noncorresponding points), Panum's areas (corresponding areas) and cyclopean projection.

Corresponding points are paired points, one in each retina, which when stimulated give rise to a percept of common visual direction. In normal binocular vison, if the retinal images stimulating these paired points contain similar content, cortical integration of the resultant impulses will occur, resulting in a single composite percept. If the retinal images stimulating these paired points contain dissimilar content and crossing borders, cortical integration of the resultant impulses is not possible and either retinal rivalry or suppression of one set of impulses will occur. Normally, foveal centers contain such corresponding points and give rise to a straight-ahead direction, the *principal visual direction.* All other paired corresponding points are located on the retina in relation to this pair at the foveal center and give rise to a visual direction in reference to the straight-ahead direction. For example, a pair of corresponding points, one in the superior temporal quadrant of the left eye and one in the superior nasal quadrant of the right eye, will give rise to common visual direction which is down and to the right of the straight-ahead direction.

Disparate points are points, one in each retina, which when stimulated do not give rise to a percept of common visual direction (the opposite of corresponding points).

Panum's areas are areas localized in the retina of one eye, any point of which, when stimulated simultaneously with a specific retinal point in the other eye, will give rise to a single fused percept if the retinal images contain similar content. Centered in a Panum's area is the corresponding point which has a directional value in common with the specific point in the other eye; that is, the other of the paired corresponding points. Surrounding this corresponding point in a Panum's area are a number of disparate points. Thus a Panum's area contains a corresponding point and a number of disparate points, but the disparate points give rise to direction close to that of the centered corresponding point.

If the visual directions resulting from stimulation of the disparate points around the corresponding point are not too dissimilar, cortical integration of the impulses from each eye for images of a single object point is possible. If the directions from stimulation of the two eyes by images of a single object point differ too much, fusion is no longer possible and physiological diplopia results. Now the image of each eye from the single object point will be localized in two distinct and separate directions. The borderline of how great a difference in direction can be cortically tolerated with fusion still occurring, and when cortical integration is not possible with diplopia occurring, defines the limits of Panum's areas. The areas are oval, longer in the horizontal dimension and are smallest in the fovea, becoming gradually larger in the peripheral retina.

Cyclopean projection refers to spatial localization of a binocularly perceived visual sensation with reference to an imaginary, single, mental eye, the cyclopean eye, which is located between the two real eyes. The cyclopean eye represents a composite hypothetical visual perception area for the two eyes and serves as a center for directionalization, each retinal point on the cyclopean eye representing a pair of corresponding points. Hence a line of visual direction from a retinal point on the cyclopean eye through its nodal point indicates the visual direction which results when a pair of corresponding points in the two eyes is stimulated. The diagrammatic representation of visual directions from the cyclopean eye thus serves as a means of interpreting or demonstrating percepts that result from binocular stimulation.

In strabismus, one eye deviates from fixation by a given amount and the images of the object of fixation do not fall simultaneously on the foveæ of the two eyes. Since one fovea normally contains corresponding points mated with the other fovea, and since the image of the object of fixation in the deviating eye is not centered on the fovea but is located elsewhere, the images of the object of fixation will not fall within Panum's areas, and cortical integration—sensory fusion—

of these impulses is not possible. In the absence of sensory fusion, diplopia will result unless suppression of the impulses from the deviating eye takes place. What is true for the images of the object of fixation is also true for the images of nonfixated objects in the binocular field of vision and, in instances of large deviations, for the images of all objects in the binocular field of vision; that is, all objects in the binocular field of vision would be perceived as double.

Since the deviating eye is not directed toward the object of fixation, its fovea will be stimulated by the image of some other object. Thus, centered on the fovea of the two eyes are dissimilar images, one from the object of fixation and one from a nonfixated object. As previously stated, the two foveæ contain corresponding points, and these two dissimilar images, which are physically located in space at different sites, will therefore be subjectively localized in space in the same direction. They will be perceived in a visual direction corresponding to the straight-ahead direction of the fixating eye. The same type of retinal stimulation is true for images of other nonfixated objects, and in instances of larger angles of strabismus all corresponding points and corresponding areas will be stimulated by dissimilar images arising from two objects in the binocular field of vision. The simultaneous directionalization of these two dissimilar images in the same visual direction is aptly called *visual confusion*. The alternative to confusion response is the suppression of impulses from one eye.

In strabismus, then, corresponding points and areas are stimulated by nonfusable dissimilar images, resulting in visual confusion, while disparate points, outside of corresponding areas, are stimulated by similar images, resulting in diplopia. This is the opposite of normal retinal stimulation, in which similar images fall on corresponding areas for objects located in the haplopic or singleness horopter (the physical correlate in space of the horizontal dimension of Panum's areas).

The problem of spatial interpretation confronting a strabismic patient may be avoided by closing one eye, by ignoring or suppressing the undesirable impulses from the deviating eye, or by developing another pattern of visual direction (anomalous correspondence).

It is possible to acquire the sensory adaptation of suppression during youth, when visual functions are still in a developmental process and flexible. The suppression response is most intense for the fovea of the deviating eye because the fovea normally possesses the best visual acuity, because its image would be seen superimposed on the image of the fixated object, the object of maximum cortical attention, and because the foveal area enjoys the largest cortical representation. The image on the fovea of the deviating eye is both the more clearly seen and the more undesirable of the unwanted images. To block it from consciousness, impulses to a relatively large area in the visual cortex must be inhibited.

If suppression begins in early life, involves only one eye (unilateral or monocular strabismus), and is present a significant period of time, it interferes both with the normal development of visual acuity and with the maintenance of the level of visual acuity already developed. This results in the reduced or retarded vision referred to as amblyopia ex anopsia (or suppression amblyopia).

Hence it is the percept of diplopia and the confusion in unilateral strabismus of early onset which provide the stimulus for suppression, and it is the suppression, when prolonged, which is considered responsible for the amblyopia.

Anisometropic Amblyopia. The stimulus for suppression in uncorrected anisometropia (without strabismus) is quite different. In this condition, binocular fixation is present and corresponding points and Panum's areas are stimulated by similar images from the same object. Since corresponding areas are stimulated by similar images arising from the same object, the stimulus to inhibition or suppression is not diplopia or confusion. Instead, in clinically significant, uncorrected anisometropia, the stimulus to inhibition of central impulses is the relative difference in blur of the central retinal images.

For any given fixation distance, retinal images of one eye will be in relatively better focus than those of the other eye. Should the visual cortex integrate the images of the fixation object into a composite percept, it might be expected that the resulting visual acuity would be worse than that derived from the eye with the better retinal focus. The image of the object of fixation from the eye with the worse retinal focus would interfere with cortical interpretation of the impulses originating from the other eye. For a given fixation distance, one eye may provide 20/100 and the other eye 20/20 visual acuity. Cortical integration of the two images may then be expected to result in a binocular visual acuity of 20/50. In actuality, though, that does not occur. Binocular visual acuity in such an instance would be 20/20; that is, it would be the same as the acuity derived from the eye with the better retinal focus.

The central retinal impulses from the eye providing the worse visual acuity appear to be inhibited, so that under binocular conditions they do not hamper or weaken the acuity provided by the other eye. If the anisometropia remains uncorrected and central impulses from the more blurred eye continue to be inhibited, the development of acuity is retarded. This is especially so if one eye is constantly suppressed.

Amblyopia resulting from uncorrected anisometropia usually is less severe than that found in strabismus. If both anisometropia and strabismus occur together, amblyopia ex anopsia tends to be more severe than that found in strabismus without significant anisometropia.

Some writers (Duke-Elder, 1949, and Gibson, 1955) differentiate between the suppression found in strabismus and the suppression found in uncorrected anisometropia, referring to the former as *active suppression* and to the latter as *passive suppression.* The implication is that in strabismus a deeper and more intense suppression is required to eliminate diplopia and confusion than is required in anisometropia to ignore a blurred image.

Amblyopia of Extinction and Amblyopia of Arrest. Amblyopia ex anopsia may be subdivided into two types: amblyopia of extinction and amblyopia of arrest (Chavasse, 1939).

Amblyopia of extinction refers to deterioration or loss of central visual acuity relative to that previously attained. The loss is considered recoverable through corrective training procedures at any age.

Amblyopia of arrest refers to reduced central vision attributed to failure of development, faulty development or retarded development caused by constant suppression or disuse during the so-called developmental years. If left unattended after the developmental years (to the age of 6 or 7), normal development is no longer considered possible, and thus normal visual acuity will not and cannot be attained.

According to the amblyopia of arrest concept, the normal development of central vision is dependent upon the continued use of the fixation reflex and upon the continued cortical reception and interpretation of the central impulses. Should this not occur, the maximum possible central vision is that which was attained at the onset of the inhibition or disuse, which in turn is related to the age of onset.

Normal development of vision is still possible if corrective measures are instituted during the developmental or formative years, but the visual reduction will become permanent if the condition is ignored beyond that time.

As an example, a child with a history of constant unilateral strabismus demonstrates 20/100 acuity in the deviating eye. The age of onset indicates that acuity at that age is normally 20/60 and that vision for the patient's present age should be 20/30. The deterioration of vision from 20/60 (that present at the age of onset) to 20/100 represents the amblyopia of extinction component of the visual reduction. This loss can be corrected if effective training is carried out, so 20/60 vision should be achieved. The further improvement of acuity from 20/60 to 20/30 (normal for the age) will be possible because the patient is still in the developmental years. If the patient is past the developmental years, however, 20/60 will be the best attained. The arrested development has been allowed to become permanent. The difference in visual acuity between 20/30 and 20/60 represents the amblyopia-of-arrest component of the visual impairment for the patient's present age. In later life, the amblyopia-of-arrest component will be the difference between 20/20 and 20/60.

Although the Chavasse concept of amblyopia of arrest does not always hold true, it is borne out to the extent that it is uncommon to restore vision to a sharp and easy 20/20 in an eye which has been amblyopic for many years and with a history of early onset.

There is no question regarding improvement in vision; the question concerns the degree or amount of improvement. Generally, in long-standing amblyopia ex anopsia of early onset, the best attainable vision is between 20/25 and 20/50. Such improvement is frequently possible with proper treatment even in adults. On occasion, 20/20 may be obtained, but unfortunately such improvement is the exception, not the rule.

Naylor and Wright (1959) found the greatest improvement in esotropic amblyopes when onset was between the ages of 2 and 5, and less improvement when onset was before the age of 2. Maggi (1959) also concludes that the age of onset is of prime importance for prognosis and that the angle of strabismus and the age when treatment starts is of lesser importance.

The fact that the extent of improvement is frequently to 20/30 or 20/40, with an occasional 20/25 or 20/20, in patients past the developmental years, indicates that the arrested development is partially reversible or that the acuity attained at onset is better than was believed.

In reference to amblyopia of extinction, the earlier the age of onset, the more rapidly and profoundly will the attained vision be lost. After vision has been fully developed, amblyopia of extinction is less likely to occur.

Chavasse (1939), Worth (1921) and Duke-Elder (1949) state that onset of strabismus after the age of 6 will not result in amblyopia ex anopsia, that vision in the deviating eye, once fully developed, will not be significantly reduced. However, in their study, Naylor and Wright mention amblyopia in which the age of onset is between the ages of 5 and 10, which would indicate that amblyopia ex anopsia can develop even when the age of onset is past the "plastic" years.

Additional evidence is the common clinical experience of a relapse in acuity after achieving an improvement. This frequently occurs when there is a failure to follow through with a complete improvement in binocular functioning, as in the elimination of strabismus. Once acuity and fixation training ceases, if further treatment is discontinued or fails the conditions which caused the amblyopia return and amblyopia of extinction recurs. The acuity may not decrease to its original low level, but it usually does decrease.

Few will disagree that the younger the age of the onset of suppression and fixation disuse, the more rapid and greater will be the visual reduction, or that the longer corrective measures are delayed, the more difficult it will be to obtain improvement, much less normal vision. Thus the importance of immediately instituting corrective training procedures and providing the proper spectacle correction cannot be overstressed. Prompt attention to the visual problem may prevent the occurrence of amblyopia or, should it have already occurred, it may provide rapid and complete recovery. Unnecessary delays and neglect will lead to a slower rate of improvement and only partial recovery.

To provide proper care in the early stages of a visual condition which could lead to amblyopia, it is necessary that the problem be detected and diagnosed. Visual examinations at preschool ages should be performed routinely. At such young ages, visual problems are most responsive to treatment because anomalous visual habits have not had sufficient time to become permanently fixed and thus are more easily reversed. Further, the child is still in the formative years and normal development can be more readily attained.

CHAPTER 6

The Incidence and Relationships of Amblyopia

Many factors influence the findings of studies on the incidence of amblyopia, so reports on this subject differ. Some of the more important variables are (1) the level of acuity considered to constitute amblyopia, e.g., 20/30, 20/40 or 20/50, (2) the testing technique and conditions utilized to measure visual acuity, e.g., single or multiple letter exposures, Snellen letters, dot recogniton, kindergarten charts, and so on, (3) motivation, attention and cooperation of patients, e.g., children compared with adults, or army enlistees compared with army draftees, (4) the method, if any, used in establishing the level of acuity for a given patient, e.g., what percent correct of a given number of letters of a given size would be accepted as "passing," (5) the correctness of the lens prescription worn, if any, and (6) the representative nature of the sample, e.g., whether it is a random cross section of the population or a screening of school children, office patients, clinical patients, or army inductees.

The implications of these variables are apparent except for the second point. Typically, better acuities will be found with the presentation of single isolated letters than with multiple letters, especially if the spacing between letters is relatively small. A lower incidence will therefore be found if testing is performed with the former technique. Reasons for this variation in acuity are discussed in Chapter 9.

A summary of several reports on the incidence of amblyopia is presented in Table VI. The wide range in incidence of from 1.0 to 5.64 percent indicates the significance of variations in acuity criteria, testing procedures and sample compositions.

TABLE VI *Incidence of amblyopia*

Source	Nature of Sample	Criterion	Percent Incidence
Glover and Brewer (1944)	21,466 draftees in Pennsylvania between the ages of 17 and 44	20/70 or less	3.14
Theodore et al. (1944)	190,012 inductees *previously screened* and accepted for service	20/50 or less	4.04
Agatston (1944)	2,400 consecutive draftees personally examined and screened for malingering	20/40 or less	1.8
Downing (1945)	60,000 draftees in Minnesota	20/50 or less	3.2
Irvine (1948)	10,000 Air Force officers and enlisted men at discharge	Not stated	1.0
Irvine (1948)	5,000 Air Corps personnel examined for glasses	Not stated	4.0
McNeil (1955)	Children 9 to 15 years of age examined in an English county borough as related to total estimated population in this borough of children in this age bracket (6,965)	20/30 or less	2.7

TABLE VI *Incidence of amblyopia (continued)*

Source	Nature of Sample	Criterion	Percent Incidence
Cole (1959)	10,000 consecutive patients examined in his practice in Nottingham, England	20/50 or less	5.3
Cholst, Cohen, and Losty (1962)	2,986 children, 90% 7 years of age or older, at two health centers in New York City	Not stated	4.8
Helveston (1965)	9,000 men, primarily enlistees but some selectees, between ages of 17 and 25, in Minnesota in same induction center as Downing; all amblyopes personally verified	20/50 or less	1.0
Flom and Neumaier (1966)	7,017 clinic patients at the University of California School of Optometry, Berkeley, ages 10 to 50	20/40 or less and more than one line difference between the two eyes	1.7
Flom & Neumaier (1966)	2,762 children screened in two California school districts (1,561 kindergarteners and 1,201 children in grades 1 through 6), using projected single E target	20/40 or less and more than one line difference between the two eyes	1.0
Abraham (1966)	7,225 patients examined in private practice	Less than 20/25 in one or both eyes	5.64
Woo (1968)	5,354 children ages 5 to 17 in northern and eastern Ontario, Canada, using an illiterate E and Snellen chart, all subjects examined by Woo	20/40 or less (one or more letters missed on 20/30 line considered 20/40)	3.85
		20/40 or less (less than half of the 20/30 line correct considered as 20/40)	3.2

The lower incidence figures among draftees and selectees reported by Agatston (1.8 percent) and Helveston (1.0 percent) are probably related to the special screening performed to exclude malingerers.

The report by Flom and Neumaier is based on a more representative sampling of the population, but the authors indicate that the incidence figures may be unduly low. They estimate that, in the school screening sample, 0.2 percent of the amblyopes may have been missed because single rather than multiple targets were used and that 0.6 percent of the children had undergone treatment which may have eliminated or prevented amblyopia. Adding these estimates to the 1.0 percent detected raises the incidence to 1.8 percent. In the clinical sample, Flom and Neumaier state that the incidence of 1.7 percent may be low due to the large number of visually normal persons who come to that particular clinic.

The Woo study has minimized potential error in that all patients were examined by the author, the report was based on a random sampling, multiple targets were presented, and previous treatment was unlikely.

The higher incidence figure reported by Abraham (5.64 percent) may be attributed to the bias inherent in sampling office patients and to the lower acuity criterion.

It is apparent from the foregoing that, to be meaningful, incidence figures should be stated in terms of the variables upon which they are based. This is well illustrated by the Flom and Neumaier report. In their clinical sample, if the acuity criterion was 20/30 and more than one line difference between the two eyes, the incidence increased from 1.7 to 2.3 percent; if the acuity criterion was 20/30, neglecting the requirement of more than one line difference between the two eyes, the incidence increased to 3.5 percent.

Relationships to Coexisting Visual Defects

In Table VII, an analysis is made of total samples for the incidence of amblyopia in association with strabismus, esotropia, exotropia and normal binocular fixation (no strabismus). Data averages indicate that 0.98 percent (1 in 100) of the total sample has amblyopia and strabismus, 0.77 percent (3 in 400) have amblyopia

TABLE VII *Incidence of coexisting visual defects with amblyopia in total sample*

Author	Percent Strabismic	Percent Esotropic	Percent Exotropic	Percent Nonstrabismic
Glover and Brewer (21,466 draftees), 1944	0.75	0.517	0.233	2.39
Theodore et al. (190,012 inductees), 1944	1.34	0.87 (0.26 not categorized in either esotropic or exotropic group)	0.21	2.70
Agatston (2,400 draftees), 1944	0.54	—	—	1.26
Downing (60,000 draftees), 1945	1.80	1.30	0.50	1.40
Helveston (9,000 enlistees and selectees), 1965	0.48	0.40	0.08	0.52
Average	0.98	0.77	0.25	1.65

and esotropia (excluding Agatson), 0.25 percent (1 in 400) has amblyopia and exotropia (excluding Agatson), and 1.65 percent (3 in 200) have amblyopia without associated strabismus.

Table VIII indicates the percentage of amblyopes with and without strabismus for six different sources. Data averages indicate that 38 percent of the amblyopes have strabismus and that 62 percent do not.

Based on the information in tables VII and VIII, amblyopia appears to occur almost twice as frequently without associated strabismus as with strabismus.

The type of amblyopia that occurs without strabismus but in association with high or unequal uncorrected refractive errors is referred to as *refractive* or *ametropia amblyopia*. Such refractive errors include high but equal hypermetropia, myopia or astigmatism (*isoametropic amblyopia*) and clinically significant uncorrected anisometropia (*anisometropic amblyopia*). Significant anisometropia may be considered to be that in which there is a 1.00-diopter or more difference in spherical correction between the two eyes or a 1.00-diopter or more difference in cylindrical correction. Typically, those with aniso-metropia have unilateral amblyopia, while those with high but equal refractive errors have bilateral amblyopia, usually with approximately equal visual reductions.

Isoametropic amblyopia may be attributed in part to developmental anomalies if reduced vision persists after the patient has worn correc-tive lenses for a prolonged period. The refractive error would then be associated with reduced vision, but not as a cause of it. Such cases may be more properly classified as congenital or organic amblyopia.

Anisometropic amblyopia, as previously discussed, has a suppres-sion background, and it is this portion of the refractive amblyopes that is properly included in the classification of amblyopia ex anopsia.

| TABLE VIII | Incidence of amblyopia: Strabismic vs. nonstrabismic | |

Author	Percent Strabismic	Percent Nonstra-bismic
Glover and Brewer (1944)	25	75
Theodore et al. (1944)	34	66
Agatston (1944)	30	70
Sugar (1944)	36	62
Downing (1945)	55	45
Helveston (1965)	48	52
Average	38	62

If constant unilateral strabismus is present in bilateral amblyopes with high but equal refractive errors and if vision is significantly more reduced in the deviating eye, then both congenital (or organic) am-blyopia and amblyopia ex anopsia may be involved. The same is true in the case of high but unequal refractive errors with or without strabismus.

Anisometropic amblyopia comprises almost all of those numbered in the refractive amblyopia group and occurs far more frequently than isoametropic amblyopia.

To illustrate the infrequent incidence of isoametropic amblyopia, Theodore et al. found only 67 examples among 5,129 nonstrabismic amblyopes, or approximately 1.1 percent of the nonstrabismic amblyopes. Agatston found among 20,000 draftees only 6 with bilateral amblyopia and associated abnormal refractive errors. Since anisometropia comprises almost the entire group of those with refractive amblyopia, for all practical purposes the nonstrabismic category in tables VII and VIII may be considered to apply essentially to anisometropia. Thus it may be stated that anisometropic amblyopia occurs more frequently than strabismic amblyopia. It is also apparent that almost all of the amblyopes have either strabismus or anisometropia, or both.

AMBLYOPIA IN HYPERMETROPIC
VS. MYOPIC ANISOMETROPIA

Anisometropia occurs more frequently than unilateral strabismus, and thus it is not surprising that the incidence of anisometropic amblyopia is greater than the incidence of strabismic amblyopia.

Among 1,500 consecutively examined refractive cases, Brock (1962) found that 27.8 percent of 365 myopes and 9.0 percent of 1,135 nonmyopes had significant anisometropia, or a total of 36.8 percent had anisometropia. On the basis of Brock's figures, anisometropia occurs about three times as frequently in myopic patients as it does in nonmyopic patients. The incidence of amblyopia, however, was greater among the nonmyopes: 6.6 percent of the nonmyopic anisometropes and 4.4 percent of the myopic anisometropes. Similarly, Jampolsky et al. (1955), in their study of 200 nonstrabismic anisometropes, report a greater incidence of unequal acuity as well as a greater difference in acuity in the hypermetropic anisometropes than in the myopic anisometropes.

The same trend is found among anisometropic strabismics. Brock (1952) found among 100 anisometropes that in all but four the amblyopic eye was hypermetropic. In a later report (1962), Brock found that 27 percent (14 of 52) of the myopic anisometropic strabismics had amblyopia, while 42 percent (78 of 186) of the hypermetropic anisometropic strabismics had amblyopia.

The reports of Phillips (1959) and Horwich (1964) provide further evidence that hypermetropic anisometropia is the most frequent type of anisometropia associated with amblyopia. In the Phillips study, 71 percent of 131 amblyopes had hypermetropic anisometropia (over half of which were strabismic), 14 percent had myopic anisometropia (only 1 of which was strabismic), and 15 percent had antimetropia (7 of which were strabismic). In the Horwich study, 66 percent of 51 strabismic anisometropes had hypermetropic anisometropia and 33 percent had astigmatic anisometropia. Both Phillips and Horwich point out that the eye with the higher refractive error, whether it be hypermetropia, astigmatism or myopia, is the eye with the amblyopia (and the deviating eye in strabismus). This is a well-established and unquestioned fact.

Hypermetropic anisometropia, in addition to being the most frequent cause of anisometropic amblyopia, also leads to greater visual reduction. The greater the difference in refractive error, the greater the visual reduction in the amblyopic eye, particularly in hypermetropia (Jampolsky et al., 1955).

The larger visual reduction in, and the greater incidence of, hypermetropic anisometropic amblyopia may be due to the fact that in myopic anisometropia either eye may be used for fixation, depending upon the fixation distance. In contrast, in hypermetropic anisometropia there is a strong tendency to use the same eye for all fixation distances. Also, in acquired myopia the onset is typically after the age of 6 or 7, and by that age normal and complete development of visual acuity and fixation may have taken place.

AMBLYOPIA IN ANISOMETRIC STRABISMUS

Visual acuity is frequently more severely affected if both strabismus and anisometropia are present than if either strabismus or anisometropia is present separately. Brock's study (1952) of the degree of visual impairment found in anisometropia with strabismus, compared to anisometropia without strabismus, confirms this point. He examined 200 anisometropes, 100 with and 100 without strabismus, and found that in most instances the strabismic anisometrope demonstrated the greater visual reduction.

It may well be that uncorrected anisometropia leads to strabismus. By creating an obstacle to sensory fusion and an overdominance of one eye, it may serve to weaken motor fusion reflexes and binocular fixation. If uncorrected, the eye with the more blurred image would be the eye expected to deviate.

Anisometropia is frequently found with strabismus. If it led to strabismus, it is likely that anisometropic amblyopia was present prior to the strabismus and that the visual reduction was then increased by the intensified suppression. Strabismus is generally considered to develop first, with amblyopia as a secondary involvement. In this instance, the opposite would be true.

The statistical investigation of Pistocchi and Lamberti (1962) furnishes some evidence for the related roles of anisometropia, amblyopia and strabismus. Over two thirds of those with over 5 diopters of anisometropia had amblyopia and one fourth of these also had strabismus. In those with less than 2 diopters of anisometropia, less than one fifth were amblyopic and 1 percent had strabismus.

Emphasis has been placed on the role of anisometropia as a cause of amblyopia ex anopsia because amblyopia ex anopsia is frequently referred to almost exclusively in terms of strabismus, despite the fact that statistics indicate that anisometropia is more frequently associated with amblyopia than is strabismus. In fact, if a lower visual acuity criterion were used in the surveys cited, such as 20/30, the incidence of amblyopia in anisometropia would no doubt be even higher than the present data indicate. With the lower criterion, many of the anisometropes with smaller differences in refractive error would be included. The same would not be true for strabismus because the visual reduction in strabismic amblyopia is typically more severe.

Another important consideration in anisometropic amblyopia is that, unlike strabismus, there is no cosmetic clue to its existence, and thus the condition is more likely to go unnoticed and untreated. This reinforces the point previously made that visual examinations should be routinely performed on preschool children.

AMBLYOPIA AND STRABISMUS

Analyses of the incidence of strabismic amblyopia among strabismics are presented in Tables IX and X.

An average of the five sources in Table IX indicates that 30 percent of all the amblyopes were esotropic and that 8 percent were exotropic, or that there were approximately 4 esotropes to 1 exotrope. This agrees fairly closely with the data presented in Table VII, which indicates a ratio of 3 esotropes to 1 exotrope. These data therefore indicate that amblyopia is three to four times more frequent with esotropia than with exotropia.

TABLE IX *Incidence of amblyopia with esotropia and exotropia*
(*percentage of all amblyopes*)

Author	Percentage of Amblyopes with Esotropia	Percentage of Amblyopes with Exotropia
Glover and Brewer (1944)	17	7
Downing (1945)	40	15
Helveston (1965)	40	8
Theodore et al. (1944)	22	7
Sugar (1944)	32	4
Average	30	8

That should not be construed to mean that esotropia is a more frequent cause of amblyopia than is exotropia. It means that esotropia itself occurs more frequently than exotropia and that for that reason there are more amblyopic esotropes than amblyopic exotropes.

Table X provides some information on the percentage of strabismics who have amblyopia as well as the percentage of esotropes and exotropes who have amblyopia. The figures of the four sources vary considerably and no definite conclusions can be made with the

TABLE X *Incidence of amblyopia in strabismus*

Author	Percentage of Strabismics	Percentage of Esotropes	Percentage of Exotropes
Glover and Brewer (1944)	77.8% of 207	71% of 145	80% of 62
Theodore et al. (1944)	95% of 2,652	95% of 1,732	93% of 537
Naylor and Wright (1959)	—	52% of 237	—
Flom (cited by Schapero, 1961)	30% of 179	33% of 111	25% of 68

exception that esotropes and exotropes appear to have an approximately equal incidence of amblyopia. The unaccounted for variable in these data is whether or not the strabismics were constant and unilateral and of early onset. Alternating strabismics, intermittent strabismics and strabismics of late onset would be less likely to demonstrate amblyopia, while the opposite is true of unilateral constant strabismics of early onset, whether esotropic or exotropic. Costenbader, Bair and McPhail (1948), for example, found that amblyopia seldom occurs in alternating strabismics (as would be expected) and that it occurs about three times more frequently in constant strabismics than in intermittent strabismics. Most probably, the amount of visual reduction would also be more severe in the constant strabismics than in the intermittent strabismics.

In constant unilateral strabismics, the fixation reflex of the deviating eye is completely inactive and suppression of the impulses from the eye occurs constantly. The continuous presence of these two anomalies may be considered prerequisites for the development of strabismic amblyopia. Conversely, the greater the tendency to have binocular fixation or the greater the tendency to alternate fixation, the less the chance of developing amblyopia ex anopsia.

AMBLYOPIA AND ANOMALOUS CORRESPONDENCE

Little information is available on the relationships of amblyopia ex anopsia, the type of correspondence and the type of strabismus. An analysis of Flom's data (cited by Schapero, 1961) on 111 esotropes and 68 exotropes reveals the following relationships:

1. Amblyopic esotropes tended to have anomalous correspondence (62 percent), while nonamblyopic esotropes tended to have normal correspondence (64 percent).

2. Both amblyopic and nonamblyopic exotropes had a higher incidence of normal correspondence than anomalous correspondence (76 percent in the former and 82 percent in the latter).

3. Esotropes with anomalous correspondence were divided approximately equally between those with amblyopia (46 percent) and those without amblyopia (54 percent), while esotropes with normal correspondence had a higher incidence of normal vision (77 percent nonamblyopic).

4. Exotropes, whether with normal or with anomalous corre-

spondence, had an approximately equal and high incidence of normal vision (76 percent nonamblyopic in the former and 70 percent non-amblyopic in the latter).

The data indicate that the amblyopic esotrope is more likely to have anomalous correspondence than the nonamblyopic esotrope or exotrope and that the esotrope with anomalous correspondence is more likely to have amblyopia than the esotrope with normal correspondence or the exotrope.

CHAPTER 7

The Mechanism of Amblyopia ex Anopsia

The prevailing opinion among investigators attributes the reduction or retardation of vision in amblyopia ex anopsia to the effects of disuse, inhibition or suppression, but the pathogenesis or site of involvement has not yet been determined.

Site of Involvement

Evidence in numerous reports indicates that any of four sites are affected: the retinal receptors, the lateral geniculate body, the visual cortex or the reticular formation of the brain stem. Possibly all four sites are involved, the malfunctioning of one affecting the other three. A discussion of the research on the nature of the impairment of visual functioning in amblyopia ex anopsia will provide greater insight into this condition and reveal the many complexities involved.

THE RETINA

Stiles-Crawford Effect No. 1. As a result of his work on the Stiles-Crawford effect No. 1 in amblyopia, Enoch (1957, 1959) suggested that the retinal receptors themselves may be at fault, being malorientated or tilted or having anomalies in their internal structure. The work of Campbell and Gregory (1960) and of Green (1967), however, has shown that malorientation of the receptors would result in only a minor loss of acuity. Further, Marshall and Flom (1968) raise the question that an anomalous Stiles-Crawford effect found in amblyopic eyes may be due to eccentric fixation rather than to malorientation of the retinal receptors.

Pugh (1958, 1962) hypothesizes that there may be an acquired tilting of the retinal receptors in the deviating amblyopic eye in strabismus. She reasons that light from the field of the fixation target is obliquely incident on the retinal receptors of the deviating eye, that the obliquely incident light results in a gradient of light stimulation on the retina, and that, as a consequence, the pigment granules of the pigment epithelium become rearranged or the retinal receptors tilt in accordance with the obliquity of the incident light.

Pugh's conclusion is based upon a careful analysis of the impressions of test letters furnished by amblyopic subjects. Test letters fixated by the amblyopic eye were reported to be distorted, with variations and gradations in brightness and definition. The letters appeared brighter and more clearly defined on the side corresponding to the direction of the strabismic deviation (see Figure 3). Right esotropes, for example, reported that the left side of a test letter, or the left letters of a line of letters, had better definition than the opposite side, which appeared smudged or faded. Pugh's work implies that an anomalous Stiles-Crawford effect is a fairly common occurrence in strabismic amblyopia.

Several points may be raised against Pugh's interpretation of the amblyopes' interesting impressions of test targets. Light from the area to which the visual axis of the deviating eye is directed is entering the eye normally. In strabismus, light from the area of the fixation target strikes a region of the retina which is usually suppressed. Assuming that the retinal receptors do tilt and that an anomalous Stiles-Crawford effect No. 1. does result, it is doubtful that it would result in the pronounced difference in appearance reported. Although Pugh states that all subjects had centric fixation, the effects described may be attributable to undetected eccentric fixation. The retinal site used in eccentric fixation is typically nasal to the foveal center in esotropia and temporal in exotropia. Thus, in right esotropia, if a site nasal to the foveal center is used in monocular fixation, the left

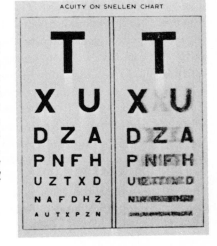

Figure 3. Appearance of the letters of an acuity chart as seen by a right amblyopic eye in right exotropia, as depicted by Pugh. The direction of clearest definition is to the left side and the direction of poorest resolution is to the right side. (*Reprinted from the* British Journal of Ophthalmology, 1962, *Volume 46, pp. 193–211, by permission of the author, editor and publisher.*)

side of the target's image (or images of targets to the left of the fixated target) will fall closer to the foveal center than the right side, which may result in the portion of the image closer to the foveal center (the left side) being seen more distinctly and with better definition than the right side.

Pugh had come to a similar conclusion in an earlier report (1951); she noticed that in amblyopia ex anopsia a disturbance in brightness sensitivity is demonstrated which may be due to a peripheral defect in the retinal receptor mechanism, as an abnormal Stiles-Crawford effect. She found, in checking stereofusion in both untreated and successfully treated amblyopia, that the illumination before the nonamblyopic eye had to be reduced to approximately 1/100 of that presented to the amblyopic eye in order to obtain balanced stereo-fusion. This was in contrast to normal eyes, in which such a difference in illumination tended to break down stereofusion.

Pupillary Light Reflex. There is some evidence that the pupillary light reflex is affected in amblyopia ex anopsia. Since the pupillomotor pathway is not considered to reach the geniculate body, such an anomaly may be the result of synaptic inhibition in the retina. Harms (1938) reached this conclusion upon finding a lowered pupillomotor response in the amblyopic eye for central stimulation as compared to the normal eye. Central retinal stimulation normally causes a more marked pupillary constriction than peripheral retinal stimulation, but the reverse was found in the amblyopic eye.

Dolénk et al. (1962) also found a difference in pupillary reaction between the amblyopic eye and the normal eye, but the difference, except for an increased latent period of contraction, disappeared after visual training.

Normally, the amount of pupillary contraction evoked by retinal illumination of one eye is the same as that evoked in that eye by retinal illumination of the other eye, assuming equal light intensities and equal dark adaptation. Also, the equal and simultaneous illumination of both eyes evokes a greater pupillary contraction from the size in the dark than is evoked by the illumination of one eye alone. However, Doesschate and Alpern (cited by Alpern et al., 1967), in a study of two amblyopes (one an alternating esotrope with an amblyopic left eye, the other a right eye amblyope without strabismus), found that the illumination of the nonfixating eye (the right eye in both instances) resulted in less pupillary contraction of the fixating (left) eye than did the illumination of the fixating eye. They also found that the equal and simultaneous illumination of both eyes resulted in no greater pupillary contraction from the size in the dark than that obtained by the illumination of the fixating eye alone.

Bárány and Halldén (1947, 1948) indicate that the central nervous system may play a part in pupillary light reflex. They found a phasic inhibition of the pupillary light reflex in normal eyes during retinal rivalry when the fovea of the nonperceiving eye was stimulated. They were also able to weaken or abolish retinal rivalry by administering drugs that depress the central nervous system.

Oxygen Level. Bietti (1950, 1955) believes that suppression in strabismus involves both the retina and the cortex, because anoxia (produced locally by compressing the eyeball and systemically by breathing air of low oxygen content) deepened suppression, whereas hyperoxia (produced locally by subconjunctival injection of oxygen and systemically by breathing oxygen) alleviated suppression.

Electroretinography. Electroretinographic studies have been performed by some investigators to examine the functioning of the receptor mechanism in amblyopia or, as Bessière et al. (1957) suggest, to differentiate between amblyopia ex anopsia and retinal disease. Some anomalies in the ERG have been reported, such as a lowered amplitude in the *b* wave (Frezzotti and Nucci, 1958), a more rounded *b* wave (Perdriel and Lods, 1963) or a diminished potential of the *a* wave proportional to the severity of the amblyopia (Dossi and Luizzi, 1962). Most reports, however, have found it to be essentially normal (Straub, 1961; Schmöger and Müller, 1964; Nawratzki, Auerbach and Rowe, 1966; Burian and Lawwill, 1966).

The major problem in utilizing the ERG has been the difficulty in isolating the ERG of the central retina. Thus the central receptor mechanism may be defective and the ERG will not reveal the abnormality. As Burian and Lawwill point out, a gross macular lesion may be present and still a normal ERG may be obtained. At present, therefore, electroretinographic studies have not pinpointed the role of the central mechanism in amblyopia ex anopsia.

Critical Fusion Frequency. Determining critical fusion (flicker) frequency (CFF) in the amblyopic eye offers another avenue for investigating the role of the retina in amblyopia ex anopsia. The efficiency or sensitivity of the retinal receptor mechanism in receiving, transmitting and terminating the flow of impulses resulting from a brief light stimulation is considered to play a significant role in determining CFF. An abnormal CFF from central retinal stimulation of an amblyopic eye could therefore be construed to indicate retinal involvement.

This approach is somewhat complicated by the many variables involved in setting up the physical stimulus condition, all of which materially affect CFF for the same retinal site. Some of these variables, as outlined by Landis (1951), are: light intensity; wavelength;

ratio between length of flash and dark period; size, shape and position of the patch of light on the retina; state of light or dark adaptation; length of time the flashing light is observed; size of test patch compared to size of pupil; brightness and hue of the surrounding test patch; and method of testing (end point when flicker ceases or when flicker begins).

As a consequence of these variables and of the different test conditions employed by investigators, the results of experiments on the CFF of amblyopic eyes are in disagreement. I. Feinberg (1956), using dark-adapted subjects, a 2-mm artificial pupil and a 1.03-degree target, found the CFF in normal eyes to be significantly higher foveally than parafoveally or peripherally. In amblyopic eyes, however, CFF was significantly reduced foveally, compared to normal eyes, while parafoveally and peripherally it was approximately the same as in normal eyes. The foveal CFF in the amblyopic eye was found to be of about the same rate as that of the more peripheral retina.

Teräskeli (1934) and Miles (1949) found the CFF in amblyopic eyes to be higher centrally and lower peripherally than that found in normal eyes. Hylkema (1956) also found CFF to be higher centrally in amblyopic eyes than in normal eyes but decreased centrally in retrobulbar neuritis (a proposed means of differentiating between amblyopia ex anopsia and retrobulbar neuritis). Weekers (1955) found central CFF to be normal or higher than normal in amblyopic eyes.

These contradictory results are largely explained by the work of Alpern, Flitman and Joseph (1960). They demonstrated that variable results will be obtained without the use of an artificial pupil— that is, by permitting pupil fluctuations to occur and thus fluctuations in the amount of light striking the retina (as did Teräskeli and Miles). Under such a test condition, the amblyopic eye may demonstrate a CFF higher, lower or equal to that of the normal eye. They also demonstrated that the central CFF of amblyopic eyes varies with the luminance level. By using an artificial pupil and testing under different levels of luminance and various states of adaptation to light, they found the central CFF in amblyopic eyes to be similar to that of normal eyes at lower levels of luminance but lower than that of normal eyes at higher levels of luminance. This variation in CFF was also correlated with visual acuity at various levels of illumination. Both varied in the same manner; that is, both CFF and visual acuity showed impairment at moderate or higher levels of retinal illumination. The latter findings would confine any defect in the receptor mechanism to the cones and would indicate that the light sense at higher levels of intensity is defective.

Although the results of the reports differ, almost all agree on one point: an alteration in central CFF occurs in amblyopic eyes, with central CFF tending to approach that of the peripheral retina or rod mechanism.

Color Vision. Since color vision is dependent upon the integrity and normal operation of the retinal receptors, receptor involvement in amblyopia ex anopsia may be reflected by anomalies in color vision. As in the studies of CFF, reports on color perception in amblyopia ex anopsia are also in conflict. In addition to the method of examination, some of the disparity may be related to the type of fixation. Frequently, fixation either is erratic or is a retinal site other than the foveal center. If it is undetected or overlooked, erroneous conclusions about the existence of anomalies in color vision may be made. Lumbroso and Proto (1963), for example, found dyschromatopsia for yellow-blue in amblyopes with paramacular or extramacular fixation but a normal color sense in those with macular eccentric and normal fixation.

Zanen and Szucs (1956) found higher central thresholds in amblyopic eyes for white and four wavelengths of the spectrum, with the greatest difference being at the long-wave portion of the spectrum. They also found diminished perception of brightness and an apparent relationship between the extent of visual reduction and the achromatic and chromatic threshold levels. Pajor and Medgyaszay (1964) and Saraux (1963) reported finding a disturbance in color sensitivity, while François and Verriest (1957, cited 1965) and Oppel (1963) found color sense to be normal. Verriest, in a more recent investigation (1963, cited by François and Verriest, 1965), concluded that color vision anomalies are observed in strabismic amblyopia only if visual acuity is markedly reduced (less than 20/200), and in such instances it is probably related to fixation defects.

Color vision defects are frequently found in congenital or organic amblyopia. In fact, testing for color vision may be considered a means of differentiating between amblyopia ex anopsia and congenital or organic amblyopia, normal color vision being indicative of amblyopia ex anopsia.

Light Sense. Thresholds of light in the light- and dark-adapted eye are dependent upon the state of sensitivity of the cone and rod mechanisms. In amblyopia ex anopsia, the detection of abnormalities in light thresholds and in light discrimination therefore would indicate involvement of the receptor mechanisms.

Wald and Burian (1944) investigated absolute light threshold in the dark- and light-adapted amblyopic eye with a circular patch of light and found the thresholds to be normal centrally and peripherally in both the dark- and light-adapted state. On the basis of their results, it was concluded that a distinction exists between the light sense and the form sense and that, since the former is normal, an anomaly in cortical interpretation of form is present in amblyopia ex anopsia.

Despite the fact that Wald and Burian reported only on absolute thresholds of light, their report has been frequently cited to support the conclusion that in amblyopia ex anopsia all aspects of the light sense are normal. More recently, however, evidence has indicated that some aspects of the light sense are not normal. Much of this evidence is based upon the fact that form perception, or visual acuity, is dependent upon the discrimination of luminance differences in the retinal image.

The investigations of Ludvigh (1941, 1942, 1950), E. F. Miller (1954, 1955) and Grosvenor (1957) indicate that luminance difference thresholds are higher for amblyopic eyes than for normal eyes at higher levels of illumination but not at lower levels of illumination. Lawwill and Burian (1966) found in functional amblyopia that contrast requirements for amblyopic eyes were similar to those for normal eyes at low background luminances, but at high background luminances the contrast requirements increased while in normal eyes they decreased.

Ludvigh found a greater tendency for the impairment of light difference sensitivity when the test was confined to central stimulation; when peripheral stimulation was involved, sensitivity was the same as for normal eyes.

Both Miller and Grosvenor used bar-shaped targets instead of the circular targets used by Wald and Burian, and Miller found that amblyopic eyes continued to show a decrease in luminance threshold as the slit was increased in width beyond that demonstrated by normal eyes (in other words, after the normal eyes had reached a plateau). Miller believes that in amblyopia ex anopsia inhibition of summation fails at the fovea, which results in a more pronounced spreading of impulses to adjacent neural elements. This in turn affects luminance difference thresholds, with the central retina behaving as does the peripheral retina in the normal dark-adapted eye.

Miller's interpretation is supported by Flynn's evidence (1967) that spatial summation in the central field of the light-adapted amblyopic eye was greater than normal and similar to that found in the normal periphery. Luminance thresholds were also found to be abnormally high centrally.

Luminance thresholds normally decrease with an increase in target size up to the limit of the receptive field center. Further increase in target size produces no further decrease in luminance thresholds and may even result in an increase because of the effect of lateral inhibition on the antithetical region surrounding the center of the receptive field. Since receptive fields are smaller centrally than peripherally, less summation occurs centrally.

Flynn concludes that the greater spatial summation found centrally in amblyopia ex anopsia indicates an enlargement of the central receptive fields. If the ganglion cell of the retina is considered to be the fundamental neural unit determining receptive field size, an increase in the size of the center of the receptive field may indicate a breakdown in the inhibitory boundary of the receptive field. The loss of or decrease in inhibitory activity would result in an increase in the effective size of the central receptive field and hence an increase in spatial summation.

Also bearing on light sensitivity in amblyopia ex anopsia is the work of Alpern, Flitman and Joseph (1960), who found CFF and visual acuity to be normal at low levels of illumination but not at high levels. The variation in acuity with the state of light adaptation and illumination has been found by many investigators and will be discussed more fully in Chapter 9.

Dark Adaptation. Another approach to the examination of light sensitivity in amblyopia ex anopsia is to study the speed of dark adaptation and the dark-adaptation curve. Szucs (1957) found the speed of dark adaptation in amblyopic and normal eyes to be the same, but amblyopic eyes showed higher terminal thresholds. Oppel and Kranke (1958) found the final dark-adaptation values in eyes with strabismic amblyopia to be the same as those in normal eyes, but they found a significant difference in adaptation between amblyopic and normal eyes in the region of the Kohlrausch's bend (the bend or kink in the adaptation curve normally produced by the increased sensitivity of the rods). In over two thirds of the cases studied, the bend occurred earlier and at higher thresholds in the amblyopic eye than it did in the normal eye. These findings were considered by Oppel and Kranke to be an indication that the cone apparatus in strabismic amblyopia was reduced in sensitivity and effectivity while the rod apparatus was normal.

Saiduzzafar and Ruben (1962, 1963) studied the course of dark adaptation in normal eyes and in eyes with strabismic amblyopia by determining absolute light thresholds as a function of time. Initially, no significant difference in thresholds was found, but after the thirteenth minute of dark adaptation the amblyopic thresholds were significantly higher, which indicates reduced sensitivity of the scotopic mechanism. In a second phase of the same experiment, visual acuity thresholds (or resolution capacities) were measured as a function of background illumination. The greatest difference in visual acuity thresholds between normal and amblyopic eyes was found when the background illumination was at photopic levels.

The results of a study by Flynn (1968) indicate threshold defects in both the cone and the rod phases of the dark-adaptation curve. The monocular absolute threshold of dark adaptation was measured over a 30-minute period on the normal and amblyopic eyes of 10 children with strabismic amblyopia. The study was initially performed during the early phase of pleoptic treatment and again six months later. A large circular grid target, subtending an angle of 11 degrees on the retina, was used to offset the influence of eccentric fixation, which was present in 4 subjects. The amblyopic eyes demonstrated statistically significant elevated thresholds which began immediately and persisted throughout the cone phase and part of the rod phase of the curve. The increased threshold was more pronounced when measured the first time but remained present when measured after six months of continued training. The rate of threshold change and the cone-rod transition time were similar to those for normal eyes.

To summarize, the preponderance of evidence presented by reports on pupillary light reflex, CFF and luminance difference and dark-adaptation thresholds indicates that light sensitivity is impaired in amblyopia ex anopsia. Whether these functions are affected by central or by peripheral influences remains unresolved.

LATERAL GENICULATE BODY

Of the possible sites involved in amblyopia ex anopsia, the lateral geniculate body has received little attention. Recent reports by Wiesel and Hubel (1963, 1965), however, offer information which bears indirectly but importantly on possible changes in both the lateral geniculate body and the visual cortex in amblyopia ex anopsia. They performed a series of experiments on newborn kittens and adult cats to determine the effects of various degrees of light deprivation on the morphology and physiology of cells in the visual pathway. Light deprivation was accomplished by suturing the eyelids, by suturing the nictitating membrane over the cornea, and by placing a translucent plastic contact lens over an eye. In each instance, form vision was excluded. The experiments were performed monocularly and binocularly on visually inexperienced kittens and on visually experienced adult cats. In monocular visual deprivation, all visually inexperienced kittens, regardless of the manner in which light stimulation was reduced, showed definite histological changes in the layers of the lateral geniculate body fed by the deprived eye, although their receptive fields appeared essentially normal. These cells appeared to be either retarded in development or atrophic. The severity of the histological changes varied directly with the amount of light deprivation, its duration and the age at which it was initiated. The translucent contact lens caused the least amount of change, and light deprivation by lid suture on adult cats caused no change. Essentially the same results were obtained on binocular lid closure experiments. Cells of other structures in the visual pathway appeared normal upon histological examination.

These results are in some disagreement with previous experiments involving binocular light deprivation in that no changes in the lateral geniculate body were found in some (Goodman, 1932; Chow, 1955), while in others (Brattgård, 1952; Chow, Riesen and Newell, 1957; Riesen, 1960; Rasch et al., 1961) changes were found in the retinal cells. Hubel and Wiesel point out that these experiments involved binocular, rather than monocular, light deprivation and that, had the cells of the lateral geniculate bodies been compared to normal cells, changes might have been detected.

Of further interest are the responses found in kittens who, after several months of light and form deprivation in one eye, were allowed to use the deprived eye with the originally exposed eye closed. In every instance, the kittens behaved as if blind, and even after prolonged use of the deprived eye they evidenced little recovery of vision. Cells in the striate area remained uninfluenced by stimulation of the originally deprived eye and continued to favor strongly the originally exposed eye; cells in the lateral geniculate body showed no evidence of recovery.

In humans who have strabismic or anisometropic amblyopia, normal light stimulation is present and thus the effect of light deprivation itself does not apply. More closely related to the experimental conditions are congenital cataracts, a condition in which light deprivation is present from birth. Even with successful surgical elimination of the cataract and with a normal-looking fundus, normal vision is not attainable; even after prolonged treatment, vision frequently remains poor. This is especially so if surgical treatment is not instituted until after the age of 5 or 6. One may speculate that a similar reaction has taken place; that is, that a retardation of development or an atrophy of cells in the lateral geniculate body receiving impulses from the deprived eye, together with cortical disuse, is responsible for the lack of improvement of vision.

In none of the experiments did the fully developed cat show ill effects from light deprivation. Only during the first three months of a kitten's life did Hubel and Wiesel find adverse reactions. Thus, once the visual pathways were fully and normally developed, they remained intact even when not in use for prolonged periods of time.

A similar reaction appears to take place in humans for corresponding ages. Juler (1921), for example, found that recoverable vision in children with unilateral traumatic cataract appeared to vary with the age at which the cataract was incurred. Examination of the corrected vision in the affected eye was conducted several years after successful surgery was performed. No child who developed a lenticular opacity at an age younger than 6½ attained vision better than 20/120, whereas all children who developed the condition after that age attained 20/40 or better. Conclusions about light deprivation causing visual loss in these cases must be moderated, however, by the influence of the coexisting factor of prolonged cortical disuse.

THE VISUAL CORTEX

The visual cortex is considered by many to be either the single site of involvement in amblyopia ex anopsia or at least the primary site, with other regions secondarily affected. A great deal of evidence, both clinical and experimental, supports this view.

Visual Acuity: Binocular vs. Monocular. In determining visual acuity in an amblyoscope with the nonamblyopic eye alternately occluded and not occluded, Pugh (1954) found that with normal correspondence a majority of patients demonstrated better visual acuity with the nonamblyopic eye occluded but that the same was not true for subjects with anomalous correspondence. She believed that her experiment provided evidence that, in strabismus with normal correspondence, the site is in the visual cortex, while in anomalous correspondence, where directional anomalies are present, the site is in the photoreceptors of the fovea. Similarly, von Noorden and Leffler (1966) found that in strabismic amblyopia the amblyopic eye demonstrated better acuity for letters on a distant chart under monocular conditions than binocular conditions. This was attributed to an increase in inhibition in the amblyopic eye under binocular conditions, a reaction likened to an exaggeration of the normal inhibitory mechanism in binocular retinal rivalry.

Occlusion Amblyopia. The occurrence of occlusion amblyopia is another indication of cortical involvement. In this condition, the non-amblyopic eye, occluded in the treatment of amblyopia ex anopsia, itself develops amblyopia and fixation anomalies while acuity and fixation improves in the nonoccluded eye (Hardesty, 1959; Krajevitch, 1962; Burian, 1966). The earlier in life that constant unilateral occlusion is instituted, the more likely and rapidly occlusion amblyopia develops.

The fact that this condition occurs especially in the very young and that it is usually reversible by discontinuing or alternating occlusion gives added weight to the concept that disuse is a cause of amblyopia, that amblyopia ex anopsia develops during the developmental years, and that it is cortical in nature.

Electroencephalography. Affection of the visual cortex in amblyopia may be indicated by abnormalities in electroencephalographic recordings. This avenue of investigation has been undertaken by many researchers, and almost all of them have found irregularities, though not necessarily with the same characteristics.

Dyer and Bierman (1950, 1952) found a high incidence of abnormal wave patterns in children between the ages of 5 and 15 and a much reduced incidence in adults in the cases of strabismic amblyopia, anisometropic amblyopia and alternating strabismus. Levinson et al. (1950, 1951) found abnormalities in approximately one third of otherwise normal strabismic subjects and twice as many abnormalities in cerebral palsy victims who also had eye involvement, compared to those without eye disorders. Parsons-Smith (1953) found abnormal cortical rhythms in almost two thirds of those with congenital amblyopia or acquired amblyopia and no relationship of incidence or type of abnormal EEG to the degree or severity of amblyopia.

Photic driving (stimulation of the eye with a flashing light at frequencies which induce an alteration in the frequency of the normal alpha rhythm) is another means of using electroencephalography to determine cortical involvement in amblyopia. The alpha rhythm occurs continuously at frequencies between 8 and 12 cycles per second, as measured at the occipital cortex (Walsh, 1966). If intermittent light stimulation is within this frequency range, summation of the induced neural excitation with the alpha rhythm takes place to produce an alteration in the recorded alpha wave.

Burian and Watson (1952) found that photic driving was less easily produced when stimulating the amblyopic eye and that it was momentary, of lower voltage and less regular when produced. Parsons-Smith (1953) found no photic driving in the majority of amblyopic eyes stimulated. In children with strabismic amblyopia, J. E. Miller et al. (1961) found no significant difference in the alpha wave, in the electroencephalogram or in *monocular* photic driving between the amblyopic eye and the normal eye or between the amblyopic subjects and the normal control subjects. They did find a significant difference in *binocular* photic driving between the amblyopic subjects and the normal subjects. The amblyopic subjects drove more at the slower frequencies of 3 to 7 cycles per second and less in the range of 8 to 18 cycles per second. In contrast, the non-amblyopic subjects drove maximally at frequencies within the normal alpha range; that is, from 8 to 13 cycles per second. This difference in binocular photic driving, however, may be related to the suppression that occurs in strabismus rather than to amblyopia.

Van Balen and Henkes (1962) measured EEG when normal and amblyopic eyes were attempting to fixate and identify a stationary test target and when they were looking to the side in response to an auditory stimulus. The authors attributed the second positive deflection of the EEG to the activity of photopic and scotopic mechanisms and found evidence of activity of the photopic mechanism in normal eyes only when in attentive states. In amblyopic eyes, even in attentive states, the photopic component tended to be smaller than that of normal eyes. Suppression in amblyopia is considered by van Balen and Henkes to be similar in its effect to inattention in normal eyes. They further state that visual attention with activation of the foveal system, at the expense of the extrafoveal system, is mediated by the reticular formation of the brain stem, and thus in amblyopia there may be a loss of reticular formation activation.

Nawratzki, Auerbach and Rowe (1966), in testing the normal and amblyopic eyes of strabismic amblyopes, found a significant prolongation in the latency of the primary response (the first upward deflection), a highly variable secondary response (the following downward deflection), and a prolonged latency when a second response was recorded. The authors were careful to point out that the measured lengthening of the latency of evoked occipital response may be due not only to a cortical defect but also to a delay in retinocortical connections.

These findings agree with the measurements of perception time and blanking time performed by von Noorden and Burian (1960). They flashed a stimulus to the eye and then, at a set time interval, presented a bright flash of light intended to interfere with the perception of the first stimulus (perceptual blanking). The purpose was to determine the shortest time interval between the presentation of the first and second stimuli, in which no perceptual blanking occurred 100 percent of the time (perception time), and the longest time interval between the presentation of the two stimuli, in which perceptual blanking did occur 100 percent of the time (blanking time). Both perception time and blanking time were found to be longer in amblyopic eyes than in normal eyes. Thus the blanking flash continued to block perception in the amblyopic eye beyond the time it affected the normal eye.

Cortical Cell Responses in Kittens and Cats. Perhaps the most important information to date which reveals the working of the visual cortex when usable information is received from just one eye, or when conflicting sensory input is received from both eyes, again relates to the works of Wiesel and Hubel on newborn kittens and adult cats.

Normally, in both kittens and adult cats, the greatest majority of cells (approximately 80 percent) in the striate cortex can be driven by the stimulation of either of the two eyes, although they may demonstrate different degrees of dominance for one eye. The responses of striate cells in visually inexperienced newborn kittens showed much the same binocular interaction and receptive field organization as in adult cats, indicating that the connections for binocular interaction are present and operative at or near birth and are not dependent on visual experience for formation. If, however, one eye of a newborn kitten was constantly deprived of form and light stimulation for two or more months, its cortical cells exhibited a consistent and marked disruption or breakdown in responsiveness to stimulation of the deprived eye. Less than 1 percent of the large number of cortical cells tested could be driven by stimulating the deprived eye, and those that did fire responded abnormally.

Unlike the histological changes found in the lateral geniculate bodies, the degree of unresponsiveness was just as marked for light deprivation a translucent contact lens as it was for lid closure: the amount of light deprivation appeared unimportant in producing the disruption. The severity of this physiological anomaly was related to the age at which deprivation was instituted, being less marked if normal visual experience was present 1 to 2 months before deprivation, with no abnormalities found if it was begun after 3 months of life. In addition, cortical potentials evoked for the two eyes were decidedly unequal and a longer latency to stimulation was found for the deprived eye (similar to EEG studies on humans with amblyopia).

Much the same results were found after strabismus was surgically induced in newborn kittens (with normal form and light stimulation) or after alternate occlusion was practiced from birth. Instead of the majority of cells in the striate cortex being driven by both eyes, with a small percent driven only by the contralateral or ipsilateral eye, as is normal, a marked shift in dominance was found, with 80 percent driven by only one eye in surgically induced strabismus and 91 percent driven by only one eye in alternating occlusion. Unfortunately, in the strabismic kittens, alternation of fixation was present, which removed from consideration the possible effects of unilateral strabismus and the resulting amblyopia. The cells of the lateral geniculate bodies of the kittens were found to be normal.

Since the striate cells were always driven normally by one eye, and since receptive fields of the lateral geniculate body were found to be operative, even in the presence of developmental abnormalities, it is likely that the site of involvement was located in the connections between the lateral geniculate body and the striate area. Further, since the unresponsiveness of the cortical cells, in all instances, could only be produced in newborn or young kittens and not in adult cats, it is reasonable to conclude that the effect of an obstacle on normal binocular functioning was related both to the type of interference and to the age at which it began. Since connections were present and operative at birth, their failure to respond normally indicates that they were disrupted or weakened by the abnormal sensory stimuli, not that they failed to become established or were dependent upon visual experience for formation.

The inability to recover normal vision, or normal cortical responsiveness, demonstrates that connections once lost or abnormally developed show little tendency to become spontaneously reestablished. It is also apparent that, for the striate cell to operate normally, the binocular input to the cell derived from corresponding points of the two eyes must be composed of signals which are compatible and of equal use. Use and disuse is therefore a factor in maintaining or enhancing the normal synaptic reception of striate cells, as is the interdependence or the interrelationship of impulses arriving at the cell.

This information has important implications when related to humans who have amblyopia. It indicates that the synaptic relay to area 17 from the lateral geniculate body is blocked for the amblyopic eye, whether due to anisometropia, in which usable sensory input is derived primarily from one eye, or to strabismus, in which conflicting sensory signals are received from both eyes. It means that the age of onset and the duration of anomalous binocular input bears importantly on the severity of visual loss and on the speed and degree of visual recovery. It supports the concepts of amblyopia of arrest and amblyopia of extinction and adds further emphasis to the importance of detecting and treating these binocular anomalies at the earliest possible age. It also agrees with the fact that amblyopia ex anopsia is not likely to occur after age 6, that is, after the visual mechanism has neared complete development.

Visual Agnosia. In investigating the functioning of the visual cortex in strabismic amblyopia from the integrative approach, Burian, Benton and Lipsius (1962) employed tests requiring the completion of fragmented figures, the detection and tracing of embedded or hidden figures, form identification based on visual memory, and the visual matching of forms based on previous tactual experience. In all instances, no significant difference was noted in responses between the normal and the amblyopic eye. It was concluded that the disturbance in strabismic amblyopia was not one of visual agnosia, that the integrative and associational areas appeared intact.

Psychological Factors

From the psychological or emotional aspect, Wekstein (1949) believes that neurosis may be a cause of amblyopia. He cites reports in which hypnotism produced temporary improvement in visual acuity. Browning and Crasilneck (1957; with Quinn, 1958) and Smith, Crasilneck and Browning (1961) attempted to improve distance and near vision in suppression amblyopia by means of posthypnotic suggestion. Significant gains were found, especially in near vision, on most of the subjects, but the improvement tended to regress. The increase in vision, although temporary, was considered to reflect an emotional component in amblyopia.

In the light of past investigations, one may theorize (1) that in amblyopia ex anopsia a sequential reaction occurs which affects the normal functioning of several components of the visual pathway of the affected eye, perhaps beginning with a disruption of synapses between the lateral geniculate body and the striate cortical cells and extending to the receptor mechanism; (2) that different types of amblyopia have been grouped under the single classification of amblyopia ex anopsia without proper identification differentiation between them and that different forms of amblyopia have different sites of involvement; (3) that failures in experimental procedures and in the statistical evaluation of results have led to erroneous conclusions. Certainly, more thorough diagnosis and more precise terminology in designating different types of amblyopia would provide a clearer understanding of the nature of this condition.

CHAPTER 8

Fixational Characteristics
of Amblyopia ex Anopsia

Steady Fixation

Chapter 4 described the characteristics of the micromovements found in normal eyes attempting to fixate steadily a motionless target. Such information is helpful in analyzing the characteristics of steady fixation found in amblyopia ex anopsia, for the minute movements normally found appear highly exaggerated in this condition.

Untreated, light-adapted amblyopic eyes in unilateral strabismus exhibit marked unsteadiness characterized by frequent drifts, flicks or jerks, and nystagmoid movements (Mackensen, 1957; von Noorden and Burian, 1958; Lawwill, 1968). The degree of instability of fixation appears to be related to the type of fixation present and to the size of the area encompassing the retinal sites used on repeated attempts to fixate. It has been found more unsteady when fixation is nonfoveal (von Noorden, 1964) and when the area encompassed by fixation attempts is large (von Noorden and Mackensen, 1962). Mackensen (1957) and Lawwill (1968) found unsteadiness to be correlated with the degree of amblyopia. Lawwill also noted that the more frequently occurring and larger amplitude drift movement was associated with a fading of the acuity target, the fading being reported as drift began. Although one would expect the unsteadiness of fixation to be related to the distance from the fovea of the retinal area used for fixation, that has not yet been shown experimentally.

The anisometropic amblyope appears to demonstrate less instability than the strabismic amblyope (Matteucci, 1960); in strabismic amblyopia, fixation becomes steady or more steady when dark adapted (in contrast to pathological causes of reduced vision) or when light adapted after successful treatment (von Noorden and Burian, 1958; Mackensen, 1957). The improvement in steady fixation when dark adapted is another manifestation of the improved performance found in amblyopia ex anopsia under conditions of reduced illumination—visual acuity and CFF being other examples.

Pursuit and Saccadic Fixation

In attempting to fixate continuously a moving target or to shift fixation abruptly from one target to another, the amblyopic eye again demonstrates inaccuracies and irregularities not demonstrated by a normal eye, especially in strabismic amblyopia.

Von Noorden and Mackensen (1962), in studying pursuit fixation in normal and strabismic amblyopic eyes, found that the unsteadiness demonstrated in steady fixation becomes more accentuated in pursuit fixation. Typically, the movements were coarse and jerky and tended to disintegrate into saccadic movements at slower target speeds than did pursuit movements of normal eyes. A relationship appeared to exist between this motor performance and fixational behavior: the more remote the site of fixation was from the fovea, the coarser were the eye movements and the faster they broke down. The level of visual acuity reduction, in itself, appeared to be unrelated to the motor disturbance.

Mackensen (1957) also found pursuit movements to be jerky and nystagmoid, and he found saccadic fixation to be more unstable than steady fixation, the degree of abnormality not corresponding to the degree of amblyopia. Both Mackensen (1958) and von Noorden (1961) found that the amblyopic eye demonstrated a slower reaction time between the presentation of a stimulus and the movement of the eye than did the normal eye, particularly if the fixation target was small. Peculiarly, von Noorden and Mackensen (1962) and Hermann and Priestley (1965) reported that the sound eyes of strabismic amblyopes do not perform as steadily or as smoothly in steady and pursuit fixation as do the eyes of normal subjects.

As was the case for steady fixation, saccadic fixation improved in the amblyopic eye when dark adapted (von Noorden and Burian, 1958), but pursuit movements did not (von Noorden and Mackensen, 1962).

The precision of motor performance in amblyopia ex anopsia is thus characterized by marked deficiencies which diminish as fixation becomes central.

Eccentric Fixation

In amblyopia ex anopsia, when the amblyopic eye actively attempts to fixate under monocular conditions, the image of the object of fixation is frequently found to be positioned off the center of the fovea, a condition known as eccentric (or anomalous) fixation. This is in contrast to normal fixation, in which the image is centered on the fovea (centric fixation).

Disagreement exists over the use of the term *eccentric fixation:* sometimes it is defined as fixation in which the image of the object of fixation falls outside of the central retina. According to this interpretation, the image of the fixated object could be located anywhere within the foveal or macular area and fixation would still be considered centric. Differentiating fixation on the basis of whether the image is on the central retina or on the peripheral retina fails to indicate or to identify adequately an abnormal fixation. It is more precise to use the center of the fovea, not the central retina, as the reference point, since the central fovea is the site of stimulation in normal fixation. Such fixation is truly "centric," and any other site of stimulation is truly "eccentric," even if the image falls on the fovea but off center. This latter concept is used in this text.

Worth, Peckham, Brock and Smith were among the early investigators of this fixation defect, but it was generally neglected until interest was renewed by the work of Bangerter and Cüppers.

INCIDENCE

Statistics indicate that eccentric fixation is a fairly common occurrence in strabismic amblyopia. Brock (1951) found that 56 percent of 107 strabismic amblyopes did not demonstrate centric fixation; the greater the visual loss, the greater the degree of eccentricity. Bangerter (1953) found that 76 percent of 138 amblyopes demonstrated eccentric fixation; Harada and Hayashi (1958) found an incidence of 82 percent among 63 amblyopes, almost all of whom were strabismics with normal correspondence. Fitton (1962) reports finding an incidence of 71 percent among 99 cases of amblyopia ex anopsia; von Noorden (1960) reports finding a 44-percent incidence of nonfoveal fixation among 433 amblyopes, but believes it was a biased sample and that the actual incidence is probably lower; Scully (1961), in combining two separate studies, found among 498 unilateral esotropes a 23-percent incidence of noncentral fixation, which was more common when onset occurred before the age of 3 or if an anisometropia of more than 1.00 diopter also was present.

Understandably, figures vary with the composition of the sample, the tests utilized and the criteria employed, but the reports indicate that eccentric fixation certainly is not rare or even unusual in strabismic amblyopia. In anisometropic amblyopia without strabismus, however, it is not usually present (Priestley, 1960; von Noorden, 1964).

CLASSIFICATION

Since fixation response varies in many ways, it may be classified as follows:

I. Centric Fixation
    A. Steady
    B. Unsteady

II. Eccentric Fixation
   A. Constancy of retinal area used
      1. Fixed site
      2. Variable site
   B. Stability of motor performance
      1. Steady
      2. Unsteady or nystagmoid
      3. Wandering or aimless
      4. Afixation (absence of fixation movement)
   C. Location of site used
      1. Foveal off-center
      2. Parafoveal
      3. Paramacular
      4. Peripheral

Normal fixation is both centric and steady. The most minor abnormality is unsteady centric fixation, the image of the fixated object oscillating about the central fovea. In eccentric fixation, the same retinal area may always be used for fixation (fixed), or on test, retest or with change in fixation conditions a variety of retinal sites may be used (variable).

The stability of fixation may range from steady, or near normal, to a complete breakdown of fixational response. The angle of eccentric fixation (the angle between the foveal center and the retinal area used for fixation, subtended at the center of rotation of the eye) may vary from minutes of arc (foveal off-center) to many degrees (peripheral). Generally, the smaller the angle of eccentric fixation, the more fixed the site, the steadier the response, and the better the visual acuity.

RELATIONSHIP TO STRABISMIC DEVIATION

It is logical to conclude that the eccentric area is located nasal to the foveal center in esotropia and temporal to the foveal center in exotropia. It seems unlikely that in a fixation attempt the image of the fixated object passes through the central area to be positioned on a retinal site on the opposite side. Clinical experience tends to confirm this conclusion, but there is little in the way of statistical analysis to verify it.

Flom and Weymouth (1961) found the eccentric site to be located nasal to the foveal center in esotropia. Indicating that this type of fixational response is usual, von Noorden (1964) refers to eccentric fixation in which the site used is on the opposite side of the central area (temporal in esotropia and nasal in exotropia) as *paradoxic eccentric fixation*. Von Noorden and Mackensen (1962) found paradoxic fixation in a small percentage of esotropes, some of whom had undergone strabismic surgery.

A vertical component is also present in many eccentric fixators. The esotrope, for example, may tend to fixate with an area nasal and superior to the fovea (Von Noorden and Mackensen, 1962). According to Burian and Cortimiglia (1962), a vertical component is most frequently present when visual acuity is markedly reduced (20/200 or less).

RELATIONSHIP TO VISUAL ACUITY

A relationship exists between the angle of eccentric fixation and visual acuity. Visual acuity normally decreases with increased eccentricity of retinal stimulation. Hence, the larger the angle of eccentric fixation, the more remote from the central fovea is the retinal site used for fixation and the poorer is the expected visual acuity. If acuity is only slightly reduced—say, to 20/50—the site used for fixation must be relatively close to the foveal center, but if acuity is markedly reduced it is likely that the angle of eccentric fixation is relatively large. Burian and Cortimiglia (1962), for example, found angles of 5 to 20 degrees with acuities of 20/100 to 20/200 in two thirds of the eyes tested; when acuity was 20/50 or better, none of the eyes showed an angle of eccentric fixation larger than 3.5 degrees.

Flom and Weymouth (1961) found that the visual acuity of amblyopic eyes with eccentric fixation correlated closely with the normal expected acuity for the eccentric retinal site used in fixation. The low acuity found in this sample of amblyopic eccentric fixators could thus be attributed primarily to the eccentric area stimulated and the low acuity it normally provides. Based on the data in this study, Flom (1968) * devised a simplified formula for clinical use in which the acuity can be predicted by knowing the angle of eccentric fixation,

* Personal communication

or vice versa. The formula is based on the normal expected acuity value assigned to eccentric sites in a normal retina, in terms of the minimum angle of resolution. It is expressed as:

$$MAR = EF - 1 \text{ and } EF = MAR - 1$$

where MAR is the minimum angle of resolution expressed in minutes of arc and EF is eccentric fixation expressed in prism diopters.

Evidence has been presented, however, which indicates that the decrease in visual acuity with the increase in the angle of eccentric fixation does not correspond identically with the acuity reductions found in a normal eye for the same amounts of eccentric retinal stimulation. Alpern et al. (1967) plotted the visual acuity of the amblyopic eye of 4 eccentric fixators against the degree of eccentricity and compared the resulting curve to one similarly derived from a normal eye. They found that the two curves did not superimpose but that the curve derived from the amblyopic eyes demonstrated a greater visual reduction for the same magnitude of eccentricity than did the curve derived from the normal eyes.

The visual acuity of functional eccentric fixators, whether the same as or less than that of the normal eye for the same amount of eccentric retinal stimulation, does not in itself reflect the visual acuities of the more central retinal areas or mean that a progressive improvement in acuity would be manifested by stimulation of retinal sites closer to the foveal center. Inhibitional influences may result in visual reductions in the more central retinal areas so that their acuities may be equal to or less than that of the retinal site used for fixation. Hence, even if eccentric fixation is present and the visual acuity corresponds to that of the normal eye for the same amount of eccentric stimulation, the visual acuity agreement alone does not necessarily indicate that amblyopia ex anopsia is solely an anomaly of fixation.

It has been stated that if the acuity of an eccentric fixator is only slightly reduced the angle of eccentric fixation must be relatively small. However, not all small-angle eccentric fixators show only slight reductions in acuity; the visual acuity in some instances may be considerably lower than expected. This point is demonstrated by the report of Burian and Cortimiglia (1962), who found angles of eccentric fixation ranging from 0.5 to 2 degrees in 6 out of 11 patients with a maximum acuity of 20/200.

Statistics also show that not all eyes with amblyopia ex anopsia demonstrate eccentric fixation, and the visual acuity of centrically fixating amblyopes is, of course, significantly reduced from that normally attainable.

Therefore, on the basis of markedly reduced visual acuity alone, one cannot predict with certainty the existence or magnitude of eccentric fixation. A small angle of eccentric fixation may be present or fixation may even be centric. Conversely, on the basis of small-angle eccentric fixation (or centric fixation), one cannot predict with certainty what the acuity will be. It may correspond closely to that normally provided by the stimulated area or it may be more severely reduced.

The predictability of the angle of eccentric fixation on the basis of visual acuity thus appears to be more accurate when visual acuity is mildly reduced, and the predictability of visual acuity on the basis of the angle of eccentric fixation appears to be more accurate when the angle is relatively large.

CONSISTENCY

On repeated determinations of the location of the eccentric site used for fixation, it is frequently found that the same site is not consistently used but rather that a number of sites are used which tend to cluster within a given area. This area has been found to vary in size in direct proportion to its distance from the central fovea, becoming increasingly larger as the area becomes progressively more peripheral (von Noorden and Mackensen, 1962). In peripheral fixation, the area encompassing the sites of fixation may be as large as two or more disk diameters. The relation of area size to distance from fovea indicates the increasing breakdown in stability and precision of fixation as it becomes more peripheral.

BILATERAL ECCENTRIC FIXATION

Eccentric fixation is usually a unilateral phenomenon, but it may occur bilaterally in bilateral amblyopia. Von Noorden (1963) described 2 patients who appeared to have such an organic background, and Hermann and Priestley (1965) reported 20 patients with strabismus and bilateral eccentric fixation.

ECCENTRIC FIXATION
IN ANISOMETROPIC AMBLYOPIA

Although eccentric fixation is not likely to occur in anisometropic amblyopia, the possibility should not be overlooked. Priestley, Hermann and Bloom (1963) reported 21 patients with anisometropic amblyopia associated with high unilateral amblyopia. Almost all exhibited eccentric fixation in the amblyopic eye, and some responded to treatment.

CAUSES

Eccentric fixation may be due to, or associated with, both organic and functional disorders. When due to organic disorders, a pathological process has so affected the central retina that either there is complete loss of central vision and a resulting absolute central scotoma or there is a severe reduction in central vision with the surrounding retina capable of significantly better vision. Most frequently, the central foveal area is scotomatous, forcing monocular fixation with an eccentric area.

The cause of eccentric fixation in amblyopia ex anopsia cannot be as readily explained. Many theories have been advanced to account for this perversion of the normal fixation reflex, but none has found general acceptance.

Before discussing these theories, it would be well to review the factors involved in the normal fixation reflex. The central fovea normally has three attributes which act as a stimulus for the cessation of a fixation movement or for the maintenance of the fixation response: (1) maximum or peak visual acuity, (2) the principal oculocentric direction of straight ahead and (3) a retinomotor value of zero.

The term *retinomotor value* refers to a value assigned to a retinal receptor, such as the depth and directional value, which acts to provide information of the angular extent and direction the eye must rotate in to fixate a target whose image is falling on the receptor. Since, normally, an image already falling on the central fovea requires no eye rotation for fixation, the receptors in the central fovea are assigned the value of zero. The retinomotor value is closely akin to the directional value of the retinal receptors. Thus if a nonfixated object is subjectively localized 5 degrees to the right of a fixated object and attention is directed to it to assume its fixation, the eye will rotate 5 degrees in this direction. Eye movement will then normally cease and, at cessation, the fixated target will be localized as straight ahead of the eye (not necessarily the self) and interpreted with peak visual acuity.

In eccentric fixation that is of functional origin, one or more of these three attributes either are not operating or are operating abnormally. In contrast to eccentric fixation from organic causes, in which there is typically an awareness of "looking to the side" of the fixated target in order to identify it, the functional eccentric fixator is usually unaware of his abnormal response. Five principal theories account for functional eccentric fixation.

1. Theory of Nonuse or Complete Disuse of the Fixation Reflex. This theory is especially applicable to unilateral strabismus of very early onset. In such instances, the fixation reflex has never, or only briefly, been exercised and has suffered nonuse or complete disuse until the time it is tested. It is the nonuse or disuse of the reflex pathway which causes the fixational response to be unsteady and inaccurate and which prevents the end point from becoming established. This concept is predicated on the failure to develop the normal reflex act, not on the development of an abnormal fixation response to replace the normal.

2. Depressed Central Vision Theory. Since central vision is reduced in amblyopia ex anopsia, the clue of peak visual acuity at the central fovea for the cessation and maintenance of fixation is no longer present. Central vision may be equal to that of the surrounding retina, resulting in a plateau of equal acuity, or it may be less than that of the surrounding retina. If central vision is equal to that of the surrounding area, the end point of fixation may fall anywhere within this plateau. If central vision is less than that of the surrounding retina, a site adjacent to this area which provides better resolving power will be selected for the end point.

The evidence cited for this theory is the frequent presence of a relative central scotoma for form vision. It has been detected by many investigators, who report it to range from 1 to 6 degrees in size (Brock, 1951; Gibson, 1955; W. S. Smith, 1954; Duke-Elder, 1949).

Especially pertinent is the report of Pasino and Maraini (1963), who found central scotomata only in eccentric fixators.

In keeping with this concept, the angle of eccentric fixation is related to the size and intensity of the relative scotoma because the amblyopic eye fixates with an area or areas providing the best resolving power.

Advocates of this theory include Duke-Elder (1949), Bangerter (1955), Böhme (1955) and Oppel (1960, 1962). Three objections are raised: (1) The area used for fixation is frequently far from the centrally depressed area, and thus the site used is not that which provides vision equal to or better than that of the central area. (2) The area used in eccentric fixation may be less sensitive to light than the central area. This point is based on Mackensen's (1957) determination of the light sensitivity of various regions of the retina in dark-adapted eccentric fixators. His questionable results were that the retinal site used in eccentric fixation had an even higher light threshold than that of the central scotomatous area. This may be construed to indicate that the eccentric fixation site is subject to more marked inhibition than the central area over which it is preferred and thus does not provide superior acuity to that of the central area. (3) Since regions of the retina surrounding the central depressed area would provide approximately the same visual acuity, any one of a number of retinal sites might be randomly selected on each fixation attempt, if acuity alone were the deciding factor. Yet eccentric fixators tend to demonstrate a repeatable preference for a single area (von Noorden and Mackensen, 1962).

3. *Anomalous Correspondence Theory.* This theory is advocated by Cüppers (1958, 1961, 1962), who believes that in eccentric fixation the straight-ahead visual direction is shifted from the foveal center to a new eccentric area and that this shift is related to a preexisting anomalous correspondence, which is a successive manifestation of the same adaptive process.

In anomalous correspondence, the two foveæ no longer give rise to common visual direction, the fovea of one eye corresponding directionally with an extrafoveal area of the other eye. The angular shift in straight-ahead direction from the fovea to the extrafoveal area, subtended at the center of rotation of that eye, is referred to as the *angle of anomaly.*

According to this theory, the shift in visual direction manifested under binocular conditions is eventually carried over into the monocular act. The same extrafoveal site in the amblyopic eye which demonstrates the straight-ahead direction under binocular conditions is used for fixation under monocular conditions. If that occurs, the angle of eccentric fixation is equal to the angle of anomaly. In harmonious anomalous correspondence (in which the angle of anomaly is equal to the objective angle of strabismus), the amblyopic eye would make no movement to fixate upon occlusion of the normally fixating eye. The same extrafoveal retinal site in the amblyopic eye which corresponds in visual direction with the fovea of the other eye receives the image of the fixated target under binocular conditions and is used for fixation under monocular conditions. Hence, when the fixating eye is occluded, no movement is required of the amblyopic eye to position the image of the fixated target on the retinal site used for monocular fixation.

Another interpretation of this theory is that the anomalous directional values present in anomalous correspondence influence monocular fixation in the amblyopic eye. Since the straight-ahead direction normally associated with the foveal center is lost under binocular conditions, it fails to operate effectively as a clue for the end point of fixation under monocular conditions. Thus the fixation movement is weakened and is guided by other clues—visual acuity, for example.

The difference between these two variations of the same basic concept is that in the second one the area used by the amblyopic eye for fixation need not be the same area which demonstrates the straight-ahead direction under binocular conditions; there is not necessarily a complete carry-over from the binocular act to the monocular act, but rather a tendency to influence monocular spatial values and thus to adversely affect monocular fixation.

The phenomenon of monocular diplopia, occasionally seen in anomalous correspondence, supports this theory. This phenomenon, first reported by Bielschowsky (1898), is thought to indicate that the shift of the straight-ahead direction to an extrafoveal area, present in binocular vision, persists in monocular fixation. The image of the fixated object is simultaneously directed to two locations, one derived from normal monocular directionalization and the other derived from the anomalous directionalization operative under binocular conditions.

Additional evidence is the report by Cüppers (1958) that, in 50 percent of the patients examined, the angle of eccentric fixation coincided with the angle of anomaly and that, when normal correspondence was reestablished, the angle of eccentric fixation also changed.

The research of Pasino (1962) also supports this view. He found that centric fixation tended to be related to normal correspondence and that eccentric fixation tended to be related to anomalous correspondence. Missotten and Nelis (1955) reported that 14 of 20 patients examined demonstrated correspondence between the angle of eccentric fixation and the angle of anomaly.

Maggi (1959) concluded that true eccentric fixation is found only in anomalous correspondence because of deep foveal inhibition and anomalous spatial values, while in normal correspondence fixation will always be normal if the fixation target subtends a visual angle larger than the centrally depressed area.

Further confirmation comes from the work of von Noorden and Mackensen (1962) and von Noorden (1963), who reported on patients with bilateral organic disturbances of the macula of early onset in whom they found bilateral eccentric fixation, with straight-ahead direction shifted from the foveal centers to the eccentric areas. This serves to illustrate Cüppers' point that with the proper stimulus an eccentric area may acquire the straight-ahead direction under binocular conditions and that this area will then be used for monocular fixation.

In contrast, patients with a monocular organic loss of central function did not demonstrate a shift in the straight-ahead direction from the foveal center. When fixation was attempted by the affected eye, it was realized that the eye was directed not straight to the target but to the side. The same was found in normal eyes suffering from temporary functional loss in the foveal area due to intense light stimulation. The fovea still retained the straight-ahead direction and there was an awareness of looking to the side when attempting to fixate.* This use of an eccentric area peripheral to the central scotoma in monocular

---

* This type of fixational response is called *eccentric viewing* by von Noorden and Mackensen, in an attempt to differentiate it from fixation in which the straight-ahead direction is associated with the eccentrically used area. They recommend reserving the term *eccentric fixation* for the type of fixation in which the straight-ahead direction is shifted to the eccentric site; that is, when subjectively it is felt that the eye is directed straight to the target. This recommendation is of dubious merit because it tends to confuse the meaning of eccentric fixation.

organic loss of central vision and in induced temporary loss in normal eyes may be used as an argument for the depressed central vision theory.

The anomalous correspondence theory is not without opposition. Five arguments may be raised against it.

(a) Despite reports to the contrary, few subjects demonstrate a complete correspondence between the angle of anomaly and the angle of eccentric fixation; that is, the amblyopic eye fails to make a fixation movement when the normal eye is occluded and remains in its deviated position.

Oppel (1962) found none exhibiting complete correspondence among 50 untreated strabismic amblyopes, Toselli and Bertoncini (1963) found none among 150 amblyopes, and von Noorden (1966) found 4 among 18 eccentric fixators. Typically, the amblyopic eye makes a distinct fixational movement upon occlusion of the fellow eye and reveals an angle of eccentric fixation considerably smaller than the angle of anomaly. These findings are considered by Oppel as a reaffirmation of his theory (the "preponderance theory") that the amblyopic eye fixates with the area providing the best acuity, whether it is the scotomatous area or an area adjacent to it.

Urist (1955, 1961), in analyzing strabismic amblyopes in which no eye movement was demonstrated upon occlusion of the normal eye (afixation), has not included anomalous correspondence among the characteristics. Instead, he points out such features as profound amblyopia (vision usually less than 20/200) and a large central scotoma.

(b) Eccentric fixation not only occurs in association with normal correspondence but may occur more frequently in association with it than with anomalous correspondence (von Noorden, 1966; Harada and Hayashi, 1958; Toselli and Bertoncini, 1963).

(c) Eccentric fixation may develop in the normal eye following its occlusion in the process of treating an amblyopic eye (Hardesty, 1959; Krajevitch, 1962; Hermann and Priestley, 1965; von Noorden, 1966; Burian, 1966). Urist (1961), in fact, claims that after prolonged occlusion the occluded eye may make no fixation movement.

Inducing eccentric fixation by occlusion completely eliminates anomalies in binocular vision as a causative factor and lends evidence to the disuse concept. The failure of the amblyopic eye to make a fixational movement upon covering the fellow eye may not indicate that the monocular straight-ahead value has shifted from the central fovea to a peripheral area corresponding directionally to the central fovea of the other eye, as Cüppers contends; rather, it may indicate a complete breakdown of the fixation reflex.

(d) Anomalous spatial localization is an extremely frequent accompaniment of eccentric fixation. When an attempt is made by an eccentric fixator to indicate the locus of a fixated target with a hand-held pointer shielded from view, the indicated locus almost invariably does not coincide with the true physical locus; the pointer will be directed somewhere to one side of the target, not directly to it. Since in functional eccentric fixation the end point of fixation is not at the foveal center, it may be presumed either that the retinomotor value of zero has truly shifted to the eccentric retinal site used for fixation or that the motor information about the rotation or positioning of the eye is incorrect, resulting in an erroneous impression of the position of the eye. If the eccentric retinal site used for fixation has acquired the oculocentric direction of straight ahead as well as the zero retinomotor value, the perceptual and motor information will agree and spatial localization should be correct. Because anomalous spatial localization is so characteristic of eccentric fixation as to be almost pathognomonic, it is unlikely that the eccentric site possesses both the straight-ahead direction and the zero retinomotor value. Rather, it would seem that a conflict exists between the perceptual clue and the motor clue and that accurate judgments cannot be made about how the eye is directed with respect to the target or about the location in space of the target with respect to the eye. If so, the subjective feeling of looking directly at a target does not necessarily indicate that the straight-ahead direction has shifted to the eccentric site.

In eccentric fixation caused by the monocular organic loss of central function, there is an awareness, often volunteered, of looking to the side of the target. Here, both the zero retinomotor value and the straight-ahead direction remain at the foveal center, and spatial localization remains correct too. In functional eccentric fixation, there is typically an unawareness of looking to the side and spatial localization is incorrect.

A corollary of this reaction takes place in past pointing, which is due to the recent onset of paresis in an extraocular muscle, or in short pointing, which is due to a spasm in an extraocular muscle. In attempting to fixate a gross object in the field of action of the affected extraocular muscle, localization in past pointing is farther in the direction of the displacement of the fixated target, or past the target. The reverse is true in short pointing.

One might consider this to be a special case of eccentric fixation because the eye rotates either insufficiently or excessively in the direction of the fixation target due to impairment in motility, and the image of the target is not centered on the fovea. Subjectively, it is felt that the eye has rotated correctly to assume fixation, though it has not, and anomalous spatial localization results. Interestingly, when the clue of acuity is added to the stimulus by presenting a detailed target, normal spatial localization returns.

(e) The location of the eccentric area of fixation may be altered by strabismic surgery (Ehrich, 1958; von Noorden, 1960, 1964, 1966; von Noorden and Mackensen, 1962; Toselli and Bertoncini, 1963) or may vary with the direction of gaze (Böhme, 1957; von Noorden and Mackensen, 1962). If the straight-ahead value is shifted from the central fovea to another retinal site as a result of anomalous correspondence, it would be expected that it would remain, for some time at least, uninfluenced by the change in positioning of the eye.

4. Motor Theory. This theory holds that motor factors involved in the fixation reflex are responsible for, or contribute to, eccentric fixation. It has been pointed out that fixation and fixational movements by the amblyopic eye are characteristically coarse and jerky. This is most pronounced when eccentric fixation is present (Matteucci, 1960) and when the angle of eccentric fixation is large (von Noorden and Mackensen, 1962). The reported influence of surgery and the direction of gaze on the location of the site of the eccentric area are further examples of a motor relationship. Böhme (1957) speculates that there may be a paretic component to eccentric fixation.

If a motor dysfunction plays a role in eccentric fixation, perhaps it is related in some manner to an existing sensory dysfunction, such as depressed central vision or anomalous spatial values.

The motor theory implies that motor values are altered, resulting in a shift of the zero retinomotor value away from the foveal center. The shift may be independent of a shift of the straight-ahead value or may be in association with a shift to the same area which possesses the straight-ahead value.

Smith (1950) and Ehrich (1959) believe that proprioceptive impulses significantly affect motor values. In testing spatial localization on an eccentric fixator, Smith stresses that the head should be held straight or else correct localization may be manifested instead of anomalous localization.

Many reflex pathways influence the positioning of both the head and the eye. These reflexes include the tonic labyrinthine reflex from the otolith apparatus, the statokinetic reflex from the semicircular canals, the tonic neck reflex, the visual righting reflex and proprioceptive impulses from the extraocular muscles themselves. Should there be a disorganization of these reflexes, as may result from having one eye in a constantly deviated or turned position, the motor values may be affected.

5. *Local Sign Theory.* Another possibility which may contribute to a motor anomaly is that of a loss, weakening or impairment of the local sign in the central depressed or scotomatous area of the amblyopic eye. Thus, in passing an image point across the affected central area, full appreciation of the changes in direction will not occur or will not be noticed at all.

This phenomenon was observed and utilized by Irvine (1944, 1948) to map the relative scotoma in amblyopia. He abruptly placed prisms before the amblyopic eye (the other eye being occluded) in increasing amounts until a shift in direction of the fixated target was perceived for a given base-apex orientation. The magnitude of the prism producing a just noticeable change in direction of the fixated target served as a measurement of the limit of the scotoma in the meridian of the prism.

Such an occurrence would indicate that the straight-ahead value, instead of being shifted from the foveal center and functioning at another retinal site, is lost or considerably weakened and that localization in space is gross and vague, with the entire centrally depressed area giving rise to a directionalization of an ill-defined region in space rather than the pinpoint differentiation in localization normally present for foveal receptors. This would significantly affect the motor response and the end point of fixation, as the zero retinomotor value would be correspondingly affected. Thus the loss of local sign for the receptors of the depressed central area may be responsible for eccentric fixation, not reduced central vision, or the attempt to use the area providing the best acuity.

The argument against the Cüppers anomalous correspondence theory weighs heavily against this explanation of eccentric fixation. Cüppers' theory has its greatest application when the nonamblyopic eye is occluded and the amblyopic eye fails to make a fixational movement, remaining in the deviated position. Even in this instance Cüppers may be incorrect in assuming that the same retinal area in the amblyopic eye which demonstrates the straight-ahead direction under binocular conditions in anomalous correspondence is the area used by the amblyopic eye for monocular fixation. The failure of the amblyopic eye to make a fixational movement does not in itself indicate that the binocular and monocular straight-ahead directions are associated with the same retinal area. This assumption must be verified by specific tests for the angle of anomaly and the angle of eccentric fixation. It would appear more logical to conclude that an eye's failure to make a fixational movement is due to a complete breakdown of the fixation reflex in association with severe visual reduction and prolonged disuse, as indicated by Urist.

In strabismic amblyopia, it is rare to find no fixational movement of the amblyopic eye when the normal eye is occluded. Many times no movement is made initially but with urging of attention and effort a fixational movement will be achieved.

The theory that the area providing maximum acuity is the site selected for fixation is especially applicable when the angle of eccentric fixation is relatively small and constant or when training has succeeded in reducing the angle. It is least applicable when the angle of eccentric fixation is large or variable; that is, in peripheral or wandering fixation.

None of the factors discussed—motor values, local sign, proprioception, disuse, depressed central vision—can be discounted. They may all influence eccentric fixation to some extent, for in all probability it has no single cause.

CHAPTER 9

Characteristics of Visual Acuity in Amblyopia ex Anopsia

Visual Acuity and Contour Interaction

In determining the visual acuity of the amblyopic eye in anisometropic and strabismic amblyopia, relatively poor acuity may be obtained with targets in close proximity to each other, and better acuity may be obtained with single targets or with targets remote from neighboring contours. As an example, a visual acuity of 20/200 for a line of letters may improve to 20/50 for single isolated letters. The increased difficulty in identifying targets closely adjacent to other targets is called the *crowding phenomenon* or the *separation difficulty*.

Other manifestations of this phenomenon are the ability to identify only the first and last targets of a line of targets and the demonstration of better acuity for targets widely spaced than for the same sized targets or larger targets closely spaced.

Since this is such a common occurrence, especially in strabismic amblyopia, the clinical measurement of visual acuity in amblyopia should consist of two methods: the presentation of a series of targets simultaneously, as a line of letters, and the presentation of single isolated targets. Acuity determined by the first method is called *cortical acuity, separation acuity, morphological acuity* or *line acuity;* by the second, *angular acuity* or (single) *letter acuity.*

None of these terms adequately differentiates between the two methods. *Cortical acuity* was proposed to indicate the influence of neighboring targets on cortical interpretation. *Angular acuity* was proposed to indicate that only the visual angle, free from contour interference, is involved in identification. Needless to say, both cortical interpretation and the visual angle are always involved, regardless of how acuity is determined. The most descriptive terms are *line acuity* and *letter acuity* (implying single target acuity), and they will be used here.

The crowding phenomenon is also present in normal eyes, where it is minimal, being more pronounced in anisometropic amblyopia and most pronounced in strabismic amblyopia (Stuart and Burian, 1962; Maraini, Pasino and Peralta, 1963; Pasino, Maraini and Cordella, 1963).

Flom, Weymouth and Kahneman (1963) studied the spatial characteristics of the crowding phenomenon in eyes with normal vision and strabismic amblyopia by determining the influence on near-threshold acuity of contours placed at various angular separations from a monocularly fixated acuity target. They first determined single-letter ("interaction free") acuity by altering fixation distance until judgment of the orientation of the gap in a Landolt C was 80 percent correct. They then determined at this fixation distance the percentage of correct responses when the Landolt C was surrounded by four bars tangentially arranged at a given distance from the C. The distance of the bars from the C was expressed both in terms of angular subtense and in multiples of the gap width in the C (or multiples of the minimum angle of resolution).

For both normal and amblyopic subjects, detection of the gap in the C was maximally impaired when the bars were about two gap widths from the C, and resolution was virtually unaffected when the bars were more than five gap widths from the C. As an example, if the minimum angle of resolution is 1 minute of arc (20/20), contour interaction will be greatest at an angular separation of 2 minutes of arc and virtually absent at a separation of 5 minutes of arc; if the minimum angle of resolution is 3 minutes of arc (20/60), the zone of contour interaction will be three times that of the first example, with contour interaction greatest at an angular separation of 6 minutes of arc and virtually absent at a separation of 15 minutes of arc. Thus the results of this investigation indicate that both the contour separation affording maximum effect on resolution and the size of the zone of interaction are proportional to resolution capacity, or single-letter acuity.

Similar results were reported by Stuart and Burian (1962). Employing a series of charts, each containing seven rows of seven Snellen Es with a given target interspace, and using a target size commensurate with the subject's visual acuity, they determined the target separation required to obtain a score of over 80 percent correct. The subjects tested had either normal vision (corrected, uncorrected and fogged), strabismic or congenital amblyopia, or obvious pathology (cataracts and chorioretinitis), and in all instances the size of the zone interaction increased in proportion to a decrease in visual acuity.

Flom, Heath and Takahashi (1963) have shown that the site of the loss of information due to contour interaction is at a supraretinal level. Essentially the same visual impairment in resolution was produced by momentarily exposing one eye to both a near-threshold Landolt C and to four surrounding, tangentially arranged bars, as was produced when one eye was exposed to the Landolt C and the other eye to the surrounding bars (as seen binocularly).

The mechanism of the crowding phenomenon is still undetermined, although the reports of Flom et al. (1963) and Stuart and Burian (1962), which find it to vary as a function of the level of visual acuity, indicate that it is not related or peculiar to any specific cause of reduced vision.

A possible cause of the crowding phenomenon is the instability of fixation which is more pronounced in amblyopic eyes (Adler, 1959; Flom et al., 1963; Matteucci, 1960; Matteucci, Maraini and Peralta, 1963; Maraini, Pasino and Peralta, 1963). Reports of a reduction in the crowding phenomenon in dark-adapted amblyopic eyes (Thomas and Spielmann, 1963; Matteucci et al., 1963) offer evidence to support this view. Eyes with amblyopia ex anopsia demonstrate greater fixation stability when dark adapted, an improvement which may result in a reduced separation difficulty because the amblyopic eye may be more accurately directed to a target of regard and have less tendency to waver to adjacent targets.

Further evidence is the fact that the severity of the crowding phenomenon parallels the degree of fixation instability, being least marked in normal eyes in which fixation is most steady, more marked in anisometropic amblyopia in which fixation is less steady, and most marked in strabismic amblyopia in which fixation is least steady. This parallel may indicate a relationship of visual acuity, stability of fixation and the crowding phenomenon to each other in that acuity is generally more severely reduced in strabismic amblyopia than in anisometropic amblyopia; that is, eyes with greater visual reduction demonstrate greater instability of fixation and hence greater separation difficulty.

Another explanation for the crowding phenomenon is proposed by Cüppers, who believes that it may be related to the monocular diplopia sometimes present in anomalous correspondence. If each of the simultaneously presented targets is seen as double, or if a rivalry in visual direction occurs, confusion in localization and in identification results. As evidence, Cüppers states that he has found the crowding phenomenon to be more pronounced when eccentric fixation is present (which Cüppers also attributes to anomalous correspondence) and to be more accentuated for targets arranged horizontally than vertically. However, there are several arguments against the Cüppers hypothesis. The separation difficulty has been found to be related to the degree of visual reduction; it occurs in both normal and amblyopic eyes and is exaggerated in strabismic amblyopia whether correspondence is normal or anomalous. Furthermore, the crowding phenomenon has not been consistently found to be more exaggerated for horizontally arranged targets (von Noorden, 1960; Stuart and Burian, 1962); it is present whether fixation is centric or eccentric (Maraini, Pasino and Paralta, 1963); and, lastly, monocular diplopia is not a frequent accompaniment of anomalous correspondence.

E. F. Miller (1954, 1955) and Flynn (1967) have indicated that a pronounced spreading of retinal excitation takes place in amblyopia ex anopsia, due perhaps to a breakdown in the inhibitory boundary of the receptive fields. If this occurs it could be a factor contributing to the crowding phenomenon. Flom et al. (1963) discount the contrast-reducing effects of the normal optical spread of an in-focus retinal image as a factor on the basis that such a spread is too small to account for the large zones of interaction found in amblyopic eyes.

A variation in the size of the receptive field has been proposed by Flom et al. (1963) as a possible cause of the crowding phenomenon. They reasoned that, as fixation becomes progressively more eccentric, larger receptive fields are involved, and this in turn leads not only to poorer visual acuity but also to greater contour interaction as larger target areas are encompassed by the larger receptive fields. Their hypothesis is confirmed to the extent that the crowding phenomenon is most exaggerated in strabismic amblyopia, a condition in which eccentric fixation is also most likely to occur.

An additional hypothesis to account for the crowding phenomenon is the loss of precise local sign in the affected depressed central retina. This point was mentioned in reference to the cause of eccentric fixation but may also apply to the crowding phenomenon. If the central area gives rise to a vague generalized localization, targets in close proximity would be difficult to identify because they would not be directed to specific and separate locations. This is evidenced clinically by strabismic amblyopes, who when questioned state that the targets appear jumbled or unequally spaced. The typical responses of amblyopes in identifying targets out of proper sequence, in omitting targets, or in failing to count the correct number of targets may be due to poor localization, but such responses may also be due to erratic fixation.

Visual Acuity and Illumination

The photopic mechanism appears to be impaired in amblyopia ex anopsia. Von Noorden and Burian (1959) found that when visual acuity was determined in a normally lighted room, and then retested under reduced illumination achieved through the use of a neutral-density filter, the eye with amblyopia ex anopsia demonstrated little or no reduction, or even improvement, in acuity. A normal eye, however, showed a consistent reduction in vision, and an eye with an organic disorder showed a marked reduction.

Von Noorden and Burian (1959) reported similar results if the eyes were dark adapted and then exposed to targets with rheostat-controlled background illumination. The strabismic amblyope demonstrated improved acuity at low levels of background illumination, while the normal eye at the same levels demonstrated an acuity considerably below its maximum. An eye with an organic lesion again showed an even greater departure from its maximum than the normal eye.

Since in some instances it is difficult to differentiate between organic amblyopia and functional amblyopia, the measurement of visual acuity under these two conditions of background illumination may be of assistance in the diagnosis; the organic amblyope would demonstrate a marked deterioration in acuity while the functional amblyope would not. Von Noorden and Burian suggest that such a test be performed with a #96 Kodak Wratten filter of 3.0 neutral density.

The maintenance or relative improvement of visual acuity in amblyopia ex anopsia when measured in reduced illumination may be related to fixational characteristics. If eccentric or erratic fixation is present and a retinal area other than the central fovea is stimulated, the eccentric area might perform better in reduced illumination than the pure-cone foveal center.

Some credence is offered for this possibility by the investigations of Caloroso and Flom (1967, 1969) of line visual acuity thresholds in amblyopic and normal eyes at six luminance levels. They found that vision in both the amblyopic and the normal fellow eye decreased in acuity with decreased luminance, but that the normal eye demonstrated a greater total reduction, the acuities of the amblyopic and the normal eye approximating each other at the lowest luminance level. They also found, however, that if the visual acuity in the normal eye was measured parafoveally, at a retinal location which provided the same photopic visual acuity as that of the amblyopic eye, the acuities measured at all luminance levels were similar to those obtained in the amblyopic eye. These results suggest that the amblyopic eye fixates with a noncentral retinal area and that the visual acuities found at various luminance levels are related to the normal functioning of the retinal area stimulated.

Another possible interpretation is that improved fixation in the dark-adapted state is responsible. Thomas and Spielmann (1963), for example, found a decreased separation difficulty in the dark-adapted state but no improvement in acuity when single, isolated targets were presented.

PART III

Diagnostic Procedures

CHAPTER 10

The Case History

A well-conducted case history can materially assist in revealing the expected presence of amblyopia, its possible cause, the likelihood of achieving an acuity improvement, the magnitude of that improvement, the rapidity in realizing the improvement, the permanence of the improvement and the possibility of undesirable side effects from treatment.

A number of types of amblyopia were described in Chapter 5. In many of these conditions the case history holds the key to diagnosis and prognosis. Nutritional toxic and even hysterical amblyopia may be diagnosed on the basis of case history. It may also yield important knowledge regarding strabismic amblyopia.

In the event that a report of strabismus is made, one should follow with inquiries concerning the age of onset, the mode of onset, suspected contributing factors, family history, and previous treatment and results. Such information is not always easily obtained, for parents are often vague and inaccurate about when a condition began, which eye turned at onset, and whether it was intermittent or constant. Early photographs may be helpful.

AGE OF ONSET

In constant unilateral strabismus, amblyopia ex anopsia may be expected in the deviating eye when the age of onset is established as having occurred before age 5 or 6. The earlier the age of onset, the more profound the visual loss and the poorer the fixation skills. The visual acuity present at onset may be estimated by knowing the expected acuity for various age levels.

The improvement of visual acuity to be derived from training can be approximated by comparing the age of onset to the present age. Such an approximation is based on the concept of amblyopia of arrest (not always borne out) in which the amount of vision reclaimed varies with the visual acuity at onset, the extent of time the amblyopia has existed and the age at which treatment is begun.

Should present age be past the so-called plastic or developmental years, it is less likely that acuity will be improved to 20/20. And the older the patient or the longer the duration, the more slowly the limited improvement will be achieved.

Should present age be less than 5 or 6, the acuity estimated at onset does not indicate maximum improvement. Since the child is in the developmental years, it is probable that full acuity development will be obtained in a relatively short time if proper corrective procedures are immediately instituted. So the importance of early detection and prompt treatment is apparent.

MODE OF ONSET

The outlook is more favorable if strabismus was initially intermittent or was preceded by a period of binocular fixation. Since the deviating eye once exhibited a fixational movement and since its central impulses once participated in sensory fusion, the task of restoring normal fixation and acuity is simplified and the prognosis for reestablishing sensory fusion, with the elimination of strabismus, is brighter.

The permanence of an improvement in acuity in strabismic amblyopia hinges on the elimination of the strabismus and the establishment of sensory fusion. If suppression still exists after visual acuity training has been successfully completed and is permitted to become operative again by returning to binocular stimulation in the continued presence of strabismus, the condition which caused the amblyopia will be reactivated, resulting in diminishment of the improved acuity. Hence, important considerations in arriving at a prognosis include judgments about how much vision can be reclaimed, how rapidly and how permanent improvement will be, based on the chances of eliminating the problem responsible for the amblyopia.

An added point, related both to the patient's age and to the chances of curing the strabismus, is the consideration of the possible consequences in binocular vision of attempting to improve acuity in an amblyopic eye. Procedures to improve vision usually entail occluding one eye; on occasion, upon cessation of constant occlusion, diplopia is experienced because of a breakdown in peripheral suppression. Much to the consternation of all concerned, this diplopia tends to persist if subsequent treatment is unsuccessful in eliminating the strabismus.

The possibility of causing diplopia, which cannot be eliminated, increases with the length of time occlusion is practiced, the constancy of the occlusion and the patient's age. The older the patient, the greater the risk of producing constant diplopia. In evaluating strabismus, and before embarking on a program to improve acuity, it is necessary to consider this possibility.

If the case history reveals intermittent strabismus, only a slight reduction in acuity in one eye is to be expected, and then only if the deviation primarily involves one eye and occurs frequently. If an alternating strabismus is indicated, with some preference to one eye, again only a mild reduction in vision in the nonpreferred eye is to be anticipated. If no preference has been apparent, amblyopia is unlikely.

SUSPECTED CONTRIBUTING FACTORS

Suspected contributing factors, such as serious illnesses, head injuries or abnormal births, would raise the possibility of organic involvement as a cause of strabismus and/or amblyopia, as would a family history of strabismus.

PREVIOUS TREATMENT

If previous treatment was given, an attempt should be made to learn what was done, for how long and with what results. Often, efforts to eliminate amblyopia and strabismus are token in nature with corresponding result. A characteristic reply to inquiries regarding previous treatment is, "Yes, we patched an eye for a few hours a day for a few weeks, but it didn't help." Such halfhearted training is valueless and is probably recommended mostly to appease concerned parents. An equally disturbing reply is, "No, nothing was done because our doctor told us he would outgrow it." Usually the reverse is true, the amblyopia and the strabismus becoming habitually fixed and more difficult to eliminate as they continue to exist.

A report of previous training which appears to have been conducted in a thorough and determined manner should be followed up by contacting the former doctor for information on his methods and results. If the previous training was unsuccessful and if there is no reason to believe that it was not properly administered and executed its repetition is unwarranted. If the treatment does not appear to have been properly carried out or if more effective methods can be used, some optimism remains for improvement. If the training for amblyopia enjoyed some success, even though the present acuity is much lower, it is a favorable sign because in amblyopia ex anopsia vision once present can usually be restored. Knowledge of whether or not spectacles have been worn may yield some information on the nature of the visual reduction. If no spectacles were worn and if a significant refractive error is found which does not produce normal vision, it is possible that wearing the proper lens correction alone will result in improved vision. Such improvement typically occurs in previously uncorrected high isoametropia or in anisometropia when not accompanied by strabismus.

CHAPTER 11

Visual Acuity Tests

Special Considerations

The procedures to diagnose amblyopia include several tests not otherwise conducted and a more extensive examination of some functions routinely tested. An initial step in the diagnosis of amblyopia is to determine if the *corrected* visual acuity is that which is expected for the age level. Acuity evaluation in amblyopia, however, involves factors which require special consideration. Some of these factors relate to peculiarities caused by the visual defect itself and some to the construction or composition of the test charts employed.

CONTOUR INTERACTION

In anisometropic and especially in strabismic amblyopia, contour interference between neighboring test targets can materially affect visual acuity responses. One cannot be content with testing acuity in the customary manner of presenting rows of targets or single, isolated targets.

In testing with only single, isolated letters, an incomplete assessment of acuity may be made and significant acuity reductions may go undetected. This is of special importance in examining preschool children, for that is the critical age when visual defects should be detected in order that remedial measures will provide maximum improvement in both visual acuity and binocular performance.

In most acuity test charts, the spacing between targets is inconsistent and without consideration of the crowding phenomenon. The target spacing appears to be related to the length of the line on the chart and not designed to provide a consistent intertarget space relative to target size. As a result, the relative interspacing varies from one line to the next.

Acuity evaluation with such charts unnecessarily adds to the uncertainty of the actual acuity. If the spacing in the 20/50 line is relatively greater than that in the 20/60 line, for example, more correct responses may be given for the 20/50 targets than for the 20/60 targets. Conversely, if the spacing is disproportionately decreased, the patient may fail to read the smaller letters which otherwise may be within his capability.

In reference to larger sized targets, one or at best two targets are usually available per line. Thus, if acuity is reduced to the level of 20/100 or worse, the evaluation is based on the identification of one or perhaps two letters, which in effect is measuring single-letter acuity. In this low range of acuities, there is an insufficient number of targets to measure line acuity and most acuity charts have large changes in target size from line to line, leaving gaps between which acuity cannot be determined. Commonly, the acuities shift from 20/400 (one target) to 20/200 (one or two targets) and then 20/100 (two targets). Thus with the use of such charts acuity evaluation in these ranges will be relatively gross.

Recognizing these inadequacies in existing acuity charts, Flom (1966) has designed a series of 21 slides which consider the effect of target separation, the need for more targets of the same size, and the desirability of thoroughly examining acuity in the more reduced levels as well as in the near normal levels. The series is graduated from 20/9 to 20/277 and each slide contains 25 targets of the same size (Snellen Es enclosing eight Landolt Cs) with the interletter space equal to one letter diameter (Figure 4). The line acuity is based on the identifica-

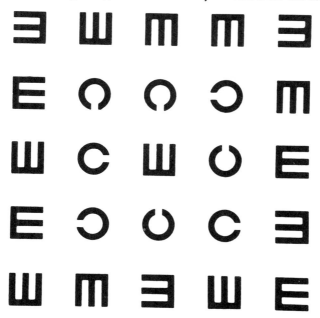

Figure 4. Flom's visual acuity test slide. The eight randomly arranged C's are the test letters and the E's provide additional contour interaction. Twenty-one slides of this target configuration cover the letter sizes from 20/277 to 20/9, the interletter spacing on all being equal to one letter diameter. (*Reprinted by permission of the Professional Press.*)

tion of the orientation of the gap in the eight Landolt Cs, all of which are surrounded by equally spaced contours.

Proper testing procedure requires that acuity be checked both with rows of targets and with single, isolated targets free from neighboring contours. This will reveal the degree to which the crowding phenomenon influences acuity. It will also provide a means of estimating expected improvements because after treatment the line acuity should improve to at least that of the single-letter acuity initially measured. Further, it will tend to reduce the possibility of erroneously believing that an acuity improvement has been achieved on retests or in the course of performing training. If it is not realized that single-letter acuity is significantly superior to line acuity, and subsequent acuities are derived from identification of single letters, an incorrect assessment of improvement will result.

There is a natural desire to measure an increase in vision after treatment and one must be careful to perform retests in the same manner and under the same conditions as those of the original test. This includes, in addition to the same testing routine and procedure of rating or scoring acuity, the same conduct on the part of the examiner; that is, not providing additional time, urging, coaxing or prompting.

VARIABILITY IN ACUITY RESPONSES

Determination of the acuity threshold level on patients with near normal vision is made with relative ease and certainty. As the minimum angle of resolution is approached, the percentage of correct responses drops rapidly from 100 to less than 50 percent, leaving little room for error in assessing acuity. The target size at which from 20 to 30 percent of the targets are missed is usually considered to be the maximum acuity, and the test is ended.

Typically, the patient will identify targets rapidly and accurately when the target size is well within his capability. When difficulty is encountered, the patient will respond more slowly and will start to make errors. With near normal vision, this takes place within a few lines of the test chart, as when a patient reads all 20/25 targets quickly and without hesitation, reads the 20/20 targets more slowly, perhaps missing one, and then reads the 20/15 targets with obvious difficulty and misses approximately one half of them.

In amblyopia ex anopsia, in contrast to normal acuity, the line acuity level at which the first errors occur—and the acuity level at which the correctness of identification decreases to less than one half of the targets—extends through a relatively large range of target sizes. The patient may correctly identify nearly the same percentage of targets for three or four lines. This leads to uncertainty in designating acuity.

One of the factors which contributes to this wide range is the construction of test charts in which the relative interletter space varies from line to line as described. Even if the relative interletter separation is maintained as a constant proportion to letter size, the first and last targets on each line, being free from contour interference on one side, are more easily identified than the middle targets. Other factors are momentary fluctuations in the steadiness of fixation, poor spatial localization and the use of Snellen letters, some of which are identified more easily than others.

The determination of single-letter acuity does not present the same degree of uncertainty because contour interference is eliminated and the influence of fluctuations in fixation is minimized. In presenting a single target by masking neighboring targets from view with a fixed-size aperture, some variation may still be experienced if the border of the mask is close enough to interact with the target. Small single targets remote from the masking border thus may be identified correctly, while

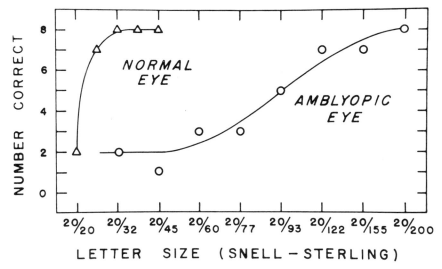

Figure 5. A plot of acuity responses for both eyes of an amblyope as tested with Flom's visual acuity test slides. Corrected for a guessing error of two letters, a correct response for seven of the eight letters corresponds to approximately 80% correct and five correct responses correspond to approximately 50%. The 80% and 50% threshold acuities obtained from the fitted curve for the amblyopic eye are about 20/135 and 20/93 respectively, and for the normal eye about 20/26 and 20/21. The flatter curve for the amblyopic eye reflects the marked variability in acuity responses. (*Reprinted by permission of the Professional Press.*)

larger targets closer to the border may be missed. Another problem in the use of an aperture of fixed size is the inability to isolate a single target when the targets are small and closely spaced.

The determination of line acuity would be greatly simplified if test charts were patterned after those of the Flom series and if the outer targets were excluded from the test. The difficulty of assessing acuity can also be reduced by graphically plotting the percent-correct responses found for each level of acuity and by fitting a curve to the plots to locate the 50-percent threshold level of visual acuity (Figure 5), a procedure recommended by Flom (1966).

BEHAVIORAL INDICATIONS OF ACUITY THRESHOLD

The behavior of the patient in identifying targets is almost as much of an indication of the acuity threshold as is the percentage of correct responses. Behavior is a particularly valuable clue when testing children.

As mentioned, as long as the angular subtense of the gap or break in the target is well within the acuity threshold, the responses are rapid, definite and unaccompanied by signs of doubt or frustration. As the task becomes more difficult, the responses characteristically become slow and hesitant and are often more in the form of query than confident answer. When the acuity threshold is approached, in addition to slowness and hesitance a child may reveal his difficulty by leaning forward, squinting, cocking his head to one side or looking at the examiner for confirmation of his answer. Other signs indicative of difficulty are attempts to look around an occluder or push it away, restlessness, and refusal to continue with the test.

When observing their child perform, parents should be cautioned not to berate the child for missing or for becoming uncooperative, and not to interject comments which reflect annoyance at the child's poor acuity or intimate that the child can see better but simply is not trying hard enough.

The examiner should also be aware that, as the test becomes difficult and the child is no longer positive of his answers, he may remark that the targets are too small and balk at further testing. At this stage, to determine if the threshold has or has not been reached, the child should be urged to try to read the "tiny" targets.

To promote confidence and continued effort, the examiner should demonstrate pleasure at a child's correct responses. This may be accomplished by reacting to a correct answer or to a show of effort with an enthusiastic remark. If the child misses, to encourage greater attention one might say, "Oh, oh, you missed that one; better look a little harder," or "I'll give you one more chance."

At a sign of balking, the examiner might switch to a different target of the same size and say, "Here's an easier one; let's see if you can get this one," or "I'll bet you can get this one if you look real hard," or "Let's see if you can get this one; I'll give you one free try."

One must always be on the alert for juvenile hysterical amblyopia, in which a child demonstrates difficulty by laboriously studying each target, responding very slowly and exhibiting great uncertainty. Since these are the usual responses to threshold-sized targets, one may erroneously conclude that maximum acuity has been reached and discontinue the test. A possible distinguishing factor is that, despite the apparent inability to interpret the targets, the percentage of correct responses remains consistently high, and, if one is patient and continues with the testing, fairly good acuity will ultimately be displayed.

LIGHT ADAPTATION AND ILLUMINATION

The state of light adaptation and target illumination may affect the acuity threshold in amblyopia ex anopsia. When the eye is dark adapted visual acuity may be better than when the eye is light adapted. When target illumination is reduced, as by viewing targets through Polaroid or neutral-density filters, acuity may remain essentially the same or may improve, a distinguishing feature from pathological or congenital amblyopia. Hence, in amblyopia testing, these two variations should be considered both from the standpoint of measuring maximum acuity and as a means of differential diagnosis.

Visual Acuity Tests

Visual acuity determination, in addition to the usual approach of identifying Snellen letters, may be performed in a variety of other ways, depending upon age, literacy and variations in test conditions. Generally, the evaluation of acuity does not present a problem except in preschool children, in whom illiteracy and lack of attention and co-operation complicate the task.

AGE TWO OR YOUNGER

In patients younger than 2, one must be content with gross estimations based upon fixation ability, the ability to locate or localize objects, or the ability to move about without running into objects.

Fixation of Light Source. Steady and pursuit fixation skills are a reflection of visual acuity, and these skills may be tested by using a light source as a fixation target, preferably one incorporated into a toy. Coaxing is usually unnecessary because the light source in the toy will attract the child's attention.

Relatively smooth and accurate fixation movements in following the light source indicate near normal vision, erratic or unsteady fixation movements indicate some visual reduction, and wandering movements or lack of fixation indicates markedly reduced vision.

A strabismus which is not cosmetically obvious may be revealed by simultaneously exposing both eyes to the light source and observing the relative positioning of the corneal reflexes. The presence of a constant unilateral strabismus would indicate reduced vision in the deviating eye.

Observation of the positioning of the corneal reflexes, as each eye fixates monocularly, provides a means of estimating the size of angle kappa in each eye, any significant difference indicating eccentric fixation in the deviating eye, which is another sign of reduced vision.

Acuity Games. Visual acuity in young patients may be approximated by using games in which forms are matched or objects of various sizes and shapes fit into corresponding depressions. Another variation is the use of beads of various sizes and colors which are picked up and dropped into a narrow-mouthed receptacle. Displaying relatively small objects (such as blocks) several feet from the patient and observing his awareness of the objects and his ability to retrieve them represents another approach to determining reduction in vision.

Reaction to Occlusion. Observing a child's reaction to occlusion serves as a means of revealing a gross reduction in vision. If the occluder is placed over one eye and the child offers little or no objection and moves freely about the room, acuity is not radically reduced. If the other eye is occluded and an immediate intense rebellion to the occluder is demonstrated or if the child is unwilling or hesitant to move about, serious visual reduction is indicated.

Optokinetic Nystagmus. When visual acuity cannot be measured subjectively, it may be determined objectively by means of optokinetic nystagmus. Acuity determined in this manner correlates fairly well with Snellen acuity (Reinecke and Cogan, 1958; Reinecke, 1959; Wolin and Dillman, 1964), and devices for producing optokinetic nystagmus are available for clinical use.

The procedure is difficult to perform on infants, however, because fixation must be directed toward the rotating drum and to be certain of the eye movements, electro-oculography should be employed. These requirements tend to limit the use of optokinetic nystagmus for acuity measurement of infants to special clinics or to investigative projects.

AGES TWO TO FIVE

If the patient is between the ages of 2 and 5, subjective tests may be attempted and are usually successful in providing accurate findings. As illiteracy is still a problem, Snellen's acuity test is impractical. In its place, a number of tests employing simplified target content are available. Such tests include the illiterate E test, the Landolt C test, Sjögren's Hand test, number tests, a variety of picture chart tests and the STYCAR tests. The method of presentation may be by wall chart, transilluminated charts, slide projection or hand-held targets.

The Illiterate E Test (tumbling E test, rotatable E test). This test is one of the most popular and widely used for acuity determination in preschool patients. The target, as the name implies, is the Snellen E presented in different directions of orientation; that is, with the limbs pointing up or down, to the right or left, or at a diagonal.

The patient is told to indicate the direction of the E verbally, by pointing with his fingers or by holding a cut out letter E in his hands and positioning it so that it matches the orientation of the target.

The test may be performed by presenting either a single E or rows of

Es. Diagonal positions are frequently omitted from the test because it is difficult for children to indicate diagonal orientation.

This "E game," as it is referred to with children, usually can be taught rather easily, even to some 2-year-olds. If difficulty is encountered, the parents can work with the child at home so that, on the next visit, he can play the game readily.

Single Es may be projected onto a screen, with all other targets masked by the aperture control of the projector, or they may be hand held. In the latter instance, one has the advantage of rotating the target to any desired orientation and also of varying the fixation distance.

A number of hand-held E tests are commercially available. Some of the ones commonly used include the Cube E Test (25), which consists of two cubes, each side of each cube containing a black Snellen E on a white background, one cube having Es ranging in Snellen acuity from 20/200 to 20/30 and the other from 20/120 to 20/20; the Hand-held E Test (27), consisting of five cards, each with a black Snellen E printed on each side, scaled for a 20-foot test distance and ranging in size from 20/100 to 20/5; and the Tumbling E Test Book (5), which consists of a ring-bound booklet of four pages of single letter Es ranging in Snellen acuity from 20/100 to 20/20. In these tests, if the fixation distance is reduced, the numerator of the Snellen fraction is the test distance. For example, if the test distance is 10 feet and letter size is marked 20/100, it becomes 10/100 (or 20/200).

Following acuity determination with single Es, the test should be continued with rows of Es because better acuity can be demonstrated with single, isolated targets than with multiple targets.

Employing rows of Es makes the test more difficult to conduct, in that a series of possible fixation targets are simultaneously presented, and one must be certain that the correct E is fixated. To ensure that the patient knows which E to fixate, the examiner, his assistant, or a parent may stand by the acuity chart and point to the E to be fixated.

For indoctrination and to instill confidence, the test should start binocularly with large single letter Es. Once the child fully understands the test, successively smaller Es are introduced until difficulty is encountered. The test is then repeated monocularly for each eye.

Responses, especially when correct, should be accompanied by praise and demonstrated pleasure in order to promote continued interest and motivation. Since a child's attention span is brief, one should proceed to the next smaller E as rapidly as possible. If the child identifies the orientation quickly and with obvious certainty, one or two correct responses per Snellen acuity level is sufficient.

Frequently, children are more cooperative and work better with closer targets, and thus it may be desirable to conduct hand-held E tests at 10 feet. Hand-held E tests are also available for testing near-point acuity (1, 9).

Landolt C Test. The Landolt C test is similar to the E test but is slightly more difficult (Jonkers, 1958) and less easily understood by preschool children. A number of Cs are presented with the gap orientated in various directions and the patient indicates the direction in which the gap is situated. The testing procedure is identical to that for the E test.

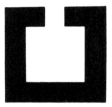

Figure 6. The Boström target. (*Reprinted from* Acta Ophthalmologica *by permission of Munksgaard and W. Nordlöw and S. Joachimsson.*)

The Boström target (26; Nördlow and Joachimsson, 1962) is a variation of the Landolt C and consists of an outline of a square with a break on one side (Figure 6). It is scaled as a Snellen letter, a 5-minute target having a 1-minute gap. Testing with this target is simpler than with the Landolt C and compares favorably with the E test.

Sjögren Hand Test. The Sjögren Hand test represents an attempt to simplify the E test. The target is a handprint including the palm and five fingers with finger separation scaled to Snellen specifications. Since the handprint is easily identified by very young patients, it is a more meaningful target. Its orientation is easier to indicate because the child's hand matches the target, and the orientation is demonstrated by holding the hand in the appropriate position. The English edition (10, 28) includes six hand-held cards, each with a single handprint ranging in size from 20/20 to 20/120. Adaptations of the test in wall chart form are also available (9).

Although this test may be more useful for testing very young children, it has the disadvantage of having only the fingers related to the Snellen standard, not the entire hand, and the relatively large palm area provides a clue to the orientation of the fingers.

Digits. The use of numbers is another approach to testing preschool children but is more appropriate for patients older than 4. In addition to this limiting feature, numbers are less easily identified than the Snellen E or Landolt C (Jonkers, 1958) and poorer acuity scores are likely to result. Testing is facilitated, however, if the patient can identify numbers as the process of indicating target orientation is eliminated.

Picture Tests. An alternate means of checking acuity, useful for preschool children from 2 to 3 years old, is by scaled pictures of familiar objects. It is simpler than tests requiring orientation identification because the child's task is merely to name the object. As with all the other tests described, it may be performed at far or near and is available in wall chart form (1, 4, 12, 16), on acuity projector slides, on hand-held targets, and in matching tests in which the child selects from an array of cutouts the one which matches the target (as in the Bailey visual perception test, 7).

In most charts, the pictures are solid, requiring recognition of the outline or shape. Consequently, such tests cannot be equated to the Snellen standard and test scores tend to be better than with any of the previously mentioned tests (Jonkers, 1958). Repetition of the same form on a smaller scale provides a memory clue and adds to the tendency toward higher scores.

In an attempt to overcome some of these shortcomings, H. F. Allen (1957) has designed a series of eight pictures in booklet form (23) which are composed of black lines with white interspaces (Figure 7). The effect of outline or shape is minimized and the spacing between the black and white areas presents a closer approximation of the Snellen specifications.

A problem in picture charts which may produce poorer scores is unfamiliarity with the test object to be identified. Most charts are composed of pictures of objects supposed to be familiar to a 2-year-old (horse, doll, house). Some test objects may be unknown, which is more likely to be true when the object is a geometric form such as a cross, square or circle. Inability to identify correctly may thus stem from unfamiliarity rather than from poor visual acuity.

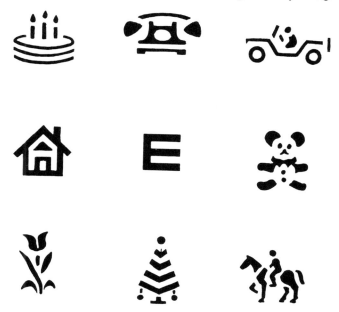

Figure 7. Picture acuity targets designed by H. F. Allen for preschool vision testing. (*Reprinted from the* American Journal of Ophthalmology *by permission of H. F. Allen and the Ophthalmic Publishing Co.*)

STYCAR Tests (*18*). Dissatisfaction with the E, Sjögren and picture tests led to the design of a series of acuity tests referred to as the STYCAR tests—Screening Tests for Young Children And Retardates (Sheridan, 1963). For ages 5 to 7, two charts were devised, one using script letters, which may be more familiar to children, the other using nine capital letters (H, L, T, C, O, X, A, V, U). These letters were considered to be the ones children learn first because they have forms resembling circles, crosses, squares and triangles, which children are able to copy by the age of 5. The letters are widely spaced, three to a line, on a 20-foot wall chart, and the child names the letters, traces them in the air with his finger or, if younger, matches them with key cards.

For the mentally retarded or for children under age 5, the test is simplified by presenting single letters at 10 feet. The letters are matched to key cards which contain nine, seven or five different letters, according to age and ability. The child points to the letter on the key card which matches the one presented by the examiner. Sheridan recommends the seven- to nine-letter key cards for 4-year-olds, the five- to seven-letter key cards for 3-year-olds, the five-letter key card for children 2½ years old and the four-letter key card (made by covering one target on the five-letter key card) for 2-year-olds.

A still simpler test for use with younger preschool children or with mentally handicapped children utilizes specially selected small toys as test objects. The toys (such as a car, doll, chair, spoon or knife) are initially presented up close to be certain the child can name them and then are held at 10 feet for identification, either by naming or by matching from a duplicate set.

AGE FIVE OR OLDER

For literate patients 5 years of age or older, the Snellen letters are used in the routine manner with the exception that both line and single-letter acuity must be determined.

Typical responses in amblyopia ex anopsia, as we have seen, are identifying letters out of sequence, cocking the head to the side when reading letters, and incorrectly counting the number of exposed letters.

On occasion, the patient may report that he can see the target to the side of the fixated target better than the fixated target, or that, to identify a target, he must direct his eye to the side of it. The first response may indicate an eccentric fixation or a depressed central area; the second, an absolute central scotoma.

A near-point acuity test should be conducted in addition to tests at 10 or 20 feet. Better vision may be found at near than at far distance (Catford, 1956), which may be due to improved fixation ability for targets close to the eyes and may be of some help in prognosis.

Supplementary Tests

One of the diagnostic problems in amblyopia is that, even though the case history, external examination, ophthalmoscopy, slit lamp biomicroscopy and visual fields yield no evidence of pathology, there still remains the possibility of undetected pathology or abnormalities.

Ophthalmometry. One of those possibilities is an anomaly of a refractive surface of the eye, especially of the anterior surface of the cornea. This may be investigated by ophthalmometry to determine if the corneal curvature is regular or irregular.

Irregularities in curvature are manifested by a distortion of the reflected mire images and by a failure of the principal meridians to be 90 degrees apart. If such irregularities are present, visual acuity should improve when a contact lens, which eliminates the curvature abnormalities, is placed on the cornea.

Pinhole Disk. A further means of checking the refractive surfaces of the eye is to measure visual acuity with a pinhole disk. Significant improvement in acuity indicates curvature or refractive irregularities.

Illumination. To assist in differentiating pathological from functional amblyopia, the acuity may be measured in both the light- and the dark-adapted state. The pathological or even the normal eye may show significant acuity reduction in the dark-adapted state and with reduced target illumination, while the eye with functional amblyopia may not (von Noorden and Burian, 1959).

Dark adaptation may be accomplished by having the patient wear dark red goggles or by confining the patient to a dark room for 15 to 20 minutes. The acuity of both the normal and the amblyopic eye is then determined through either a neutral density filter or geared Polaroid filters (22).

If a neutral density filter is used, von Noorden and Burian recommend a #96 3.00 N.D. Kodak Wratten filter. Such a filter will cause a reduction in acuity in the normal eye to about 20/40, and in an eye with pathological amblyopia to 20/40 or lower, while the acuity in an eye with functional amblyopia may remain about the same.

Two methods are available for determining visual acuity with Polaroid filters. One is to rotate the axes of the two Polaroid filters away from parallelism before the normal eye until acuity is reduced to 20/40 and then to place the filters before the amblyopic eye at the same setting. No significant change in acuity will be found in functional amblyopia compared to the acuity obtained in the light-adapted state (Kavner, 1966). In the other technique, the amblyopic eye fixates the smallest letter that can be identified in a lighted room and the axes of the Polaroid filters are rotated away from parallelism until the letter is blacked out and then toward parallelism until it reappears. The scale setting of the Polaroid filters in each instance is noted, 20 on the scale corresponding to parallelism of the axes and o when they are at right angles. According to Cowan, Bennett and Ogg (1966), if blackout is before 15 or recovery past 15, organic amblyopia is indicated; if blackout and reappearance are between 15 and 5 and 5 and 15, respectively, organic amblyopia is suspected; if blackout and reappearance are between 5 and o and o and 5, respectively, functional amblyopia is indicated.

Caution should be exercised in relying on the foregoing techniques as the sole means of differential diagnosis between pathological and functional amblyopia. Doubts have been expressed about the effectiveness of these methods in identifying the type of amblyopia present. Callahan (1961), for example, in his evaluation of the neutral-density filter test, concluded that this procedure was inconclusive in that it may fail to detect some of the organic amblyopes.

Telescopic Lens. The measurement of corrected visual acuity through a telescopic lens may be useful as a prognostic tool in indicating the likelihood of acuity improvement after treatment (Feldman, 1949; Wheeler, 1956; Fowler, 1956; D'Agostino and D'Esposito, 1962). Acuity improvement with telescopic lenses indicate that improvement may be realized with training.

CHAPTER 12

Tests of Fixation

Tests for Eccentric Fixation

Since the existence of eccentric fixation has a significant bearing on prognosis and training approach in amblyopia ex anopsia, it is necessary to test for its existence and, if present, to note all of its characteristics. These include the location of the site used and its distance from the foveal center (the angle of eccentric fixation); the area encompassed on successive attempts at fixation (fixed site vs. variable site); variations in the location of the site, if any, with change in direction of gaze; the steadiness of the response; and whether or not the principal visual direction, or subjective straight-ahead direction, is associated with the eccentric site.

A variety of tests may be used to detect eccentric fixation. Some are gross, of value mainly when the angle of eccentric fixation is relatively large, and some are precise, detecting small amounts of eccentric fixation with certainty and ease. The discussion to follow will analyze the methods commonly used.

VISUSCOPE

The Visuscope (21) is an ophthalmoscope adapted for testing eccentric fixation by the inclusion, among its accessory test targets, of a small, opaque, star-shaped target. The star pattern is seen in the light-transmitting aperture by the patient, it serves as a fixation target, and at the same time it casts a shadow of its form onto the fundus, corresponding in angular size to 40 minutes of arc (Figure 8). This test,

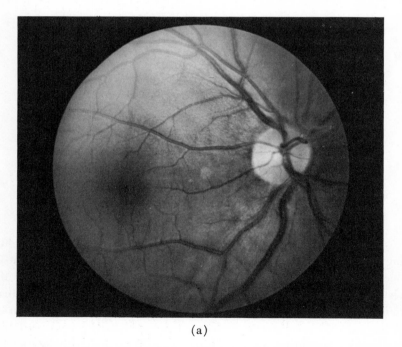

(a)

Figure 8. Photographs illustrating the fundus location of the shadow of the fixated Visuscope star target for (a) centric fixation, (b) parafoveal fixation, (c) paramacular fixation and (d) peripheral fixation.

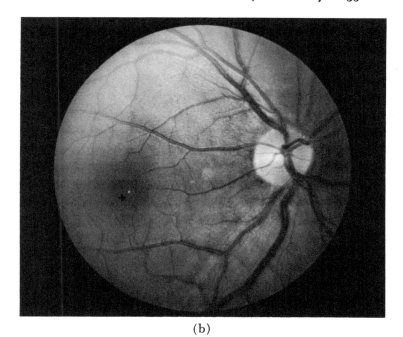

(b)

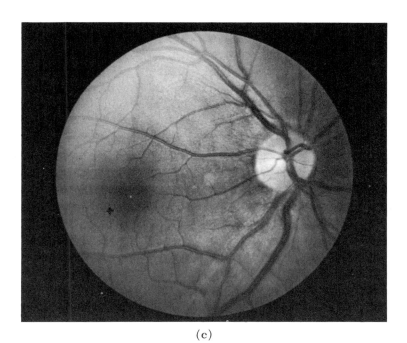

(c)

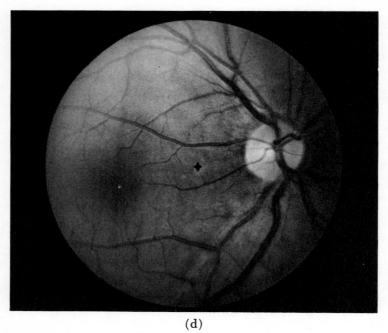

(d)

devised by Cüppers, enables the examiner to check for eccentric fixation by noting whether or not the star-shaped shadow of the fixation target is centered on the fovea.

Most foveae present a foveolar reflex, a pinpoint reflex of light from the foveal center observed during ophthalmoscopy. This reflex serves as the reference point. In normal steady fixation, the shadow covers it and is seen centered in the deeper red foveal region. In eccentric fixation, the shadow is seen either to the side of the foveolar reflex or, if no reflex is observed, not centered in the deeper red foveal area. A green filter is used in conjunction with the star target to facilitate observation and to avoid glare.

The angle of eccentric fixation—that is, the distance of the star-shaped shadow from the foveal center—may be determined by seven concentric rings which surround the star pattern and cast shadows around the shadow of the star. The rings are separated by 20-minute intervals and the angle of eccentric fixation is indicated by the number of rings between the foveal center and the shadow of the fixation target.

The test should be repeated several times and in various directions of gaze to determine if the same site is used consistently and if the direction of gaze influences the location of the eccentric site. The patient should be asked, in each instance, whether or not he feels that his eye is aimed directly at the fixation target in the instrument so that the examiner can ascertain if the straight-ahead direction is subjectively associated with the eccentric site.

Since this is a monocular test, one eye is usually occluded while the other is examined, although the test may be conducted without occlusion. Each eye should be checked to compare fixation responses, even if one eye has normal vision.

A check for a central scotoma may be made by positioning the shadow on the foveal center, with the patient looking straight ahead, to determine if it disappears or becomes fainter.

The test is one of the best available for the investigation of this fixation response because direct observation of the retinal site used for fixation is possible and steadiness and changes in the location of the site are easily observed.

Variations on this test include the use of a single E or a horizontal or vertical row of Es as shadow-casting fixation targets. The presentation of multiple fixation targets is especially valuable because saccadic fixation behavior can be observed as fixation shifts from one E to another.

PROJECTOSCOPE

A test target similar to the Visuscope star has been included among the aperture graticules available with the Projectoscope (11), another variety of ophthalmoscope. The target, the Linksz star graticule (Figure 9), is an open-center, four-pointed star pattern surrounded by two concentric circles subtending angles of 3 and 5 degrees. The open center has the advantage of exposing the foveolar reflex when normal fixation is present, simplifying diagnosis.

NEITZ EUTHYSCOPE

The Neitz Euthyscope (19), a modified ophthalmoscope, has included among its special targets an open-center, four-pointed star pattern similar to the Linksz star for the detection of eccentric fixation. It also has a target containing nine concentric circles, spaced at 0.5-degree intervals, for the measurement of eccentric fixation. The easily read dials and the thin head of the instrument make it simple to operate.

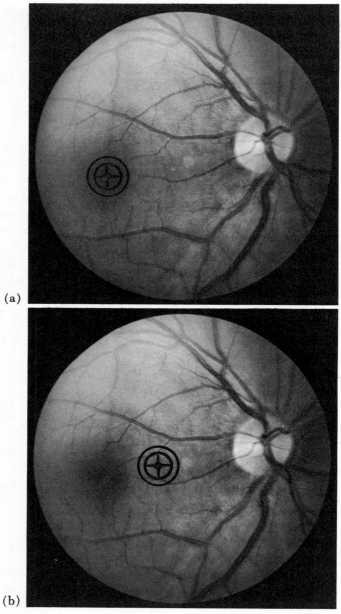

(a)

(b)

Figure 9. The shadow of the Linksz star graticule as observed with the Projectoscope in (a) centric fixation with
foveolar reflex remaining visible and (b) eccentric fixation.

As with the Visuscope, the star target of the Projectoscope or Neitz Euthyscope is used in conjunction with a green filter and the patient fixates the star while the examiner observes the fundus location of its shadow in reference to the foveal center.

OPHTHALMOSCOPE

When a Visuscope, Projectoscope or Neitz Euthyscope is not available, some ophthalmoscopes with suitable optical systems (such as the Welch-Allyn) may be adapted by placing a small opaque dot in the center of the green auxiliary filter. Another method of adapting an ophthalmoscope, especially one equipped with a bright light source, is to reduce the aperture size of the instrument so as to provide a narrow beam of light. This will furnish both a small fixation target and a small patch of light on the fundus. With the patient fixating the small light-transmitting aperture, the location of the small circle of light on the fundus (instead of a shadow) relative to the foveal center will indicate if eccentric fixation is present and, if so, its approximate magnitude. One means of reducing the aperture size is to opaque-in an infrequently used graticule on the auxiliary disk, except for a small central area.

One may use an unadapted ophthalmoscope by having the patient fixate the light of the ophthalmoscope and noting the location of the lighted area on the fundus. This, of course, is a much cruder test; the fixation target is large, as is the circle of light on the fundus, and the patient may fixate different portions of the light instead of its center, causing the light patch to be seen decentered, simulating an eccentric fixation when none may be present. By comparing the fundus positions of the light patch in the normal and in the amblyopic eye, the possibility of an erroneous diagnosis may be minimized but not eliminated. The unadapted ophthalmoscope may be used in this manner as a gross screening test during routine ophthalmoscopy, but the final diagnosis should be made with precise tests designed especially to detect eccentric fixation.

HAIDINGER'S BRUSHES

Eccentric fixation, as well as the anatomical integrity of the macular area, may be investigated through the use of Haidinger's brushes, an entoptically perceived pattern of closely packed radiating lines emanating from opposite sides of a common central point, similar in shape to an airplane propeller or a bow tie, and lying essentially in a single meridian (Figure 10). It is elicited by viewing a homogeneous field of plane polarized light, especially polarized blue light, the meridional orientation of the brushes corresponding to the axis of polarization.

The entoptically perceived, brushlike pattern is derived from the macular area, the center of the pattern corresponding to the center of the fovea. Gording (1950) believed this pattern to be related to the combined effects of the fiber layer of Henle and the yellow pigmentation in the macular area when stimulated by polarized light. Halldén (1957) concluded that it appears to be due to the interference of polarized light, with the deeper retinal layers, probably the retinal receptors themselves, acting as a radial analyzer and the fiber layer of Henle acting as a radial retarding plate.

In any event, this phenomenon is dependent upon the anatomical peculiarities of the macular area, and it may be presumed that in order to be observed the anatomical constituents (especially the retinal receptors and the fiber layer of Henle) must be normal in both structure and arrangement.

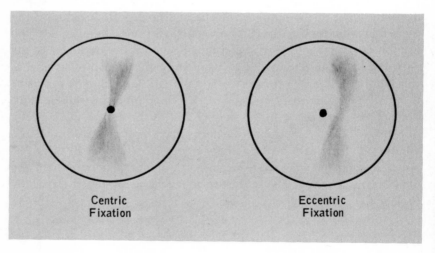

Figure 10. A diagrammatic representation of the appearance and location of the Haidinger's brushes as projected in reference to a fixation target in centric and eccentric fixation.

The test for Haidinger's brushes was originally adapted for investigating the anatomical integrity of the macular area (Goldschmidt, 1950; Murroughs, 1957) because it was thought that the inability to perceive the brushes indicated a developmental or pathological anomaly. Failure to elicit the brushes under monocular conditions is thus indicative of congenital or organic amblyopia and a poor prognosis for potential visual acuity improvement. Conversely, perceiving the brushes, while not eliminating a diagnosis of congenital or organic amblyopia, offers a more favorable prognosis for acuity improvement because the foveal and macular area now appears to be anatomically intact and capable of normal functioning.

The absence or presence of the brushes is but one of several findings in formulating a diagnosis, and no final diagnosis or prognosis should be based on this test alone. Indeed, reports have been made of instances in which the brushes were not perceived and acuity was normal or improved with training and of instances in which the brushes were perceived but acuity did not improve with training (Murroughs, 1957).

More recently, this brush effect has been put to another important clinical use, the detection and treatment of eccentric fixation. Since the brushes are derived from the central retinal area, the perceived location of the brushes will reveal the direction of the visual axis in reference to a monocularly fixated target. If the visual axis is directed precisely to the fixated target (centric fixation), the brushes will be perceived as centered about the target; if the visual axis is not directed to the fixated target (eccentric fixation), the brushes will be perceived as somewhere to the side of the target, corresponding to the point in space to which the visual axis is directed. The distance and direction of the center of the brushes (and thus the visual axis) from the fixation target indicates the retinal site used for fixation and its distance and direction from the foveal center.

To prevent retinal adaptation and to make the brush effect more noticeable, many instruments designed for this purpose employ a motor-driven rotating Polaroid filter. Since the meridional orientation of the brushes corresponds to the axis of polarization, a rotating Polaroid filter will cause the brushes to appear to rotate, simulating the effect of a rotating airplane propeller.

In some instruments, the direction of rotation of the Polaroid filter may be reversed, causing the brushes to appear to spin in the opposite direction. This reversal provides a means of verifying a response, as it should be detected by the patient.

If eccentric fixation is indicated by the localization of the brushes to the side of the target, one may determine if the oculocentric direction of straight ahead is associated with the eccentric retinal area by inquiring if it is felt that the eye is aimed directly at, or to the side of, a fixation target positioned directly in front of the fixating eye. The correctness of egocentric direction (the perceived direction in space of an object or image subjectively evaluated in reference to the self) may be determined by inquiring if it is felt that the fixated target is located directly in front of the fixating eye.

Several responses are possible, depending upon the retinal site possessing the oculocentric direction of straight ahead and the retinal site possessing the true retinomotor value of zero. It may be reported that the eye is directed straight to the target which appears to be directly in front of the eye, indicating that possibly both the zero retinomotor value and the straight-ahead direction are associated with the eccentric retinal site used for fixation; it may be reported that the eye is directed to the side of the target but that the target appears to be directly in front of the eye, indicating that both the zero retinomotor value and the straight-ahead direction are still associated with the foveal center (as occurs in a monocular, absolute, central scotoma); or it may be reported that the eye is directed straight to the target but that the target is not situated directly in front of the eye, indicating that incorrect motor information has been received as to the positioning of the eye on fixating, or possibly that the straight-ahead direction has shifted from the foveal center to the eccentric retinal site but that the zero retinomotor value has not.

An advantage of the Haidinger's brushes technique over the Visuscope or Projectoscope technique is that one need not rely on the subjective appraisal of whether the fixation target appears to be situated directly in front of the fixating eye or whether the fixating eye is directed straight at the target. The response is verified by having the patient rapidly move a pointer, positioned in front of the fixating eye, to the fixation target while constantly maintaining fixation on the target. This is done while the Haidinger's brushes are present and after their location has been established. If localization is correct, the pointer tip will be moved directly to the target while the brushes are still observed at its side. If not, the pointer tip will miss the target and will also be positioned to one side, or corrective motions will be made in an attempt to place the pointer tip on the target. The procedure should be repeated several times to test the consistency of the response and to assist in minimizing the influence of motor control of the pointer.

Correct localization indicates that both the zero retinomotor value and the principal visual direction are operative and are associated with the same retinal area, whether it is the foveal center or an eccentric retinal area. Anomalous spatial localization indicates a conflict in perceptual and motor clues and the possibility that incorrect motor information is being received as to the positioning of the fixating eye.

Examination of the influence of direction of gaze on the fixation response may be made by having the patient turn his head to the side or up or down while fixating a target positioned directly in front of the eye.

Two of the most commonly used instruments for testing (or treating) eccentric fixation by means of the Haidinger's brushes are the Coordinator (21; designed by Cüppers) and the Macula Integrity Tester-Trainer (5; designed by Vodnoy). Both are table-mounted instruments designed for testing at a near distance, and both have a motor-driven rotating Polaroid filter which is transilluminated and viewed through a deep blue filter. The target plane is adjacent and slightly closer to the eye than the Polaroid filter. The brushes under these conditions appear as a dark blue pattern against a lighter blue background.

Other instruments producing the Haidinger's brush effect which may be adapted for testing but which are used primarily for training are the Space Coordinator (21), the Neosynoptophore (21) and an attachment to the Clement Clarke synoptophore (6) which may be used independently. In the Space Coordinator, the brushes are produced by a rotating Polaroid filter closer to the eye than the target plane, requiring the projection of the brushes in space to a more distant target plane.

A complication may arise in testing for eccentric fixation with the brushes in young patients. They may fail to understand what they are to see or they may be unable to detect the brush effect. This entoptic phenomenon does not stand out boldly from the background, and close attention and scrutiny is necessary for the effect to be appreciated.

As a means of indoctrination, to minimize this difficulty the test may be conducted initially on the normal eye. By so doing with a young patient, however, one stands a greater risk of receiving the false response that the brushes are rotating about the fixation point (as was observed with the normal eye), when in fact the brushes are not perceived or are perceived elsewhere.

Another related problem, present if fixation is of the peripheral type, is that the brushes are far removed from the fixation target and, as a result, may go undetected. The inability to perceive the brushes, under these conditions, confuses the diagnosis. One cannot be certain whether the failure is due to poor insight or observation or to a histological anomaly in the macular area, with the brushes truly absent.

MAXWELL'S SPOT TEST

Another test for foveal integrity and eccentric fixation, based on an entoptic phenomenon originating from the foveal area, utilizes Maxwell's spot, which is a round dark-purplish spot, approximately 3 arc degrees in diameter, derived from the foveal area and entoptically perceived when the eye is exposed to a homogeneous blue or purple field. It was originally noticed by Maxwell in 1856 when he fixated the blue region of a prismatic spectrum. He thought it was related to the absorption of blue light by the yellow pigment in the central retina. Another interpretation, expressed by Walls and Mathews (1952), considers color receptors in the foveal cones to be responsible for the effect.

As with the Haidinger's brushes, there is agreement that the spot arises from the foveal area of the retina. It lends itself to the examination of fixation because the projected location of the spot in space indicates the direction of the visual axis in reference to a fixated target. In normal monocular fixation for a target presented in a blue or purple field, Maxwell's spot is seen centered about the target (W. R. Miles, 1948, 1949; Flom and Weymouth, 1961). In eccentric fixation, Maxwell's spot is seen displaced to the side of the fixation target by an angular amount equivalent to the amount of eccentric fixation.

The determination of the location of the spot in reference to a fixation target, usually presented at near, and the measurement of its distance from the target serve as a measure of eccentric fixation.

The test may be performed clinically by having the patient monocularly fixate a small black target on a white field which is viewed through a dichromic filter transmitting only red and blue, or by viewing a screen bathed in light projected through such a filter. Two color filters best suited to produce the purplish field are Roscoe purple No. 28 and Kodak Wratten experimental filter No. 2389.

Since Maxwell's spot fades quickly with constant exposure to the purple field, the eye should be alternately exposed to achromatic light, as may be provided by a Kodak Wratten neutral filter No. 96, density 1.5. On exposure to the purple field, Maxwell's spot is seen as a dark purple spot in the purple field; on exposure to the gray field, its afterimage is seen as a greenish spot.

As with the Haidinger's brushes, a problem may arise because young patients may be unable to distinguish the spot from its background, either because they fail to comprehend what it is they are to see or because they are not astute observers. This leads to confusion in diagnosis and prognosis because a true failure to elicit the spot indicates an anomaly in the integrity of the foveal area and a poor prognosis for subsequent acuity improvement. For purposes of indoctrination, the test may be conducted initially on the normal eye.

The Maxwell's spot test may be conducted with a commercially available testing apparatus, the Eccentric Fixation Tester Disk (24). However, it is a relatively simple matter to set up this test, the primary requirements being a lighted field with a fixation target, a purple filter and a neutral-density filter.

COMPARISON OF ANGLE KAPPA

Larger amounts of eccentric fixation may be detected by measuring angle kappa (more correctly angle lambda *) of each eye and then comparing the magnitudes.

Angle kappa is the angle between the pupillary axis (the line perpendicular to the cornea and passing through the center of the entrance pupil of the eye) and the visual axis, subtended at the nodal point. When the patient fixates a light source positioned directly below the observer's eye, the corneal light reflex is typically seen posi-

---

* The angle between the pupillary axis and line of sight subtended at the center of the entrance pupil.

tioned slightly nasal to the center of the entrance pupil (the image of the pupil formed by refraction through the cornea). The corneal light reflex is displaced nasally since, normally, the fovea is not positioned on the optic axis of the eye (or the extension of the pupillary axis) but lies templeward to it. In the act of fixating, the pupillary axis is

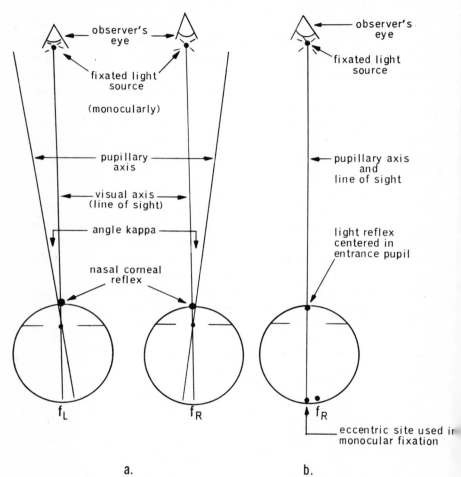

a.   b.

Figure 11. The measurement of angle kappa (lamda) with the penlight technique: (a) normal monocular fixation in the right and left eyes with equal nasal displacement of the corneal light reflex and (b) eccentric fixation in the right eye with the line of sight coincident with the pupillary axis resulting in a centered corneal light reflex and a zero angle kappa.

rotated slightly templeward, as the visual axis is directed to the fixation target, causing the corneal light reflex to be positioned on the nasal side of the center of the entrance pupil by approximately 0.5 mm. Angle kappa is designated *plus* when the light reflex is positioned nasally and *minus* when it is positioned temporally.

If fixation is normal in each eye, the angle measured in one eye is equal in sign and magnitude to the angle measured in the other eye (assuming the eyes are symmetrical). If fixation in one eye is grossly eccentric, a significant difference between the two angles will be found (Figure 11).

Penlight Technique. Angle kappa may be measured by several alternate methods. The one most frequently used employs a penlight positioned approximately 50 cm in front of the patient's fixating eye, the other eye being occluded. The examiner sights monocularly over the light source, notes the position of the corneal reflex, and estimates its vertical and lateral displacement in millimeters from the center of the entrance pupil or measures its displacement with a millimeter rule. The procedure is repeated for the other eye and a comparison is made of the two estimates or measurements in order to determine whether or not a significant difference exists. If so, eccentric fixation in the amblyopic eye is indicated.

This method is relatively gross and should be confirmed with more precise techniques before making a positive diagnosis. Failure to observe or to measure a difference in the location of the corneal reflex between the two eyes does not eliminate the possibility of the existence of an eccentric fixation of an angle smaller than can be detected by this method. This may easily occur, as a 3-degree angle of eccentric fixation results in only approximately a 0.5-mm difference in the positioning of the corneal reflexes.

Major Amblyoscope Method. An equally satisfactory method of measuring angle kappa involves the use of a major amblyoscope such as the Troposcope or synoptophore. Slides used for this purpose contain a horizontal graduated scale on a clear background with a series of fixation targets in the form of numbers, letters or familiar objects. The patient monocularly fixates the target corresponding to the zero mark on the scale, while the examiner, facing the patient, sights directly over the tube and notes the position of the corneal reflex created by the instrument's light transilluminating the target. The patient is then instructed to fixate sequentially the targets to the appropriate side of the zero mark until the corneal reflex appears centered. The target fixated on the scale when the corneal reflex is centered serves as a measure of angle kappa, which may be converted into prism diopters by knowing the focal length of the eyepiece. For the Troposcope it is 20 cm and for the synoptophore it is 15 cm. Thus, every 2-mm displacement from zero on the scale for the Troposcope and every 1.5-mm for the synoptophore is equivalent to one prism diopter. Slide 2 of the George Washington University Diagnostic Series is used with the Troposcope to measure angle kappa (Figure 12), and each fixation target on the scale is separated by 2 arc degrees. The procedure is repeated for the other eye and a comparison is made between the two measurements.

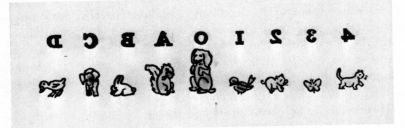

Figure 12. Slide #2 of the George Washington University Diagnostic Series, used on the American Optical Companies Troposcope for the measurement of angle kappa.

Arc Perimeter Technique. A third technique for determining angle kappa utilizes the arc perimeter. With one eye occluded, the patient steadily fixates the central target on the perimeter arc. The examiner places a penlight directly beneath his eye, monocularly sights the position of the corneal reflex from the top of the perimeter arc starting at the zero mark, and moves his eye along the arc in the appropriate direction until the reflex appears centered. The degree mark on the scale at which the penlight is positioned when the reflex appears centered is a direct measure of angle kappa. For greater accuracy, the procedure should be repeated two or three times on one eye before proceeding to the other.

BLIND SPOT TEST

This test for eccentric fixation originally proposed by Peckham (1941) necessitates plotting the blind spot of Mariotte (physiological blind spot) for each eye and noting whether or not the center of each blind spot is equally displaced from the fixation target. The blind spot is plotted in the usual manner, as on a tangent screen at a 1-meter fixation distance. An unequal displacement indicates eccentric fixation of the amblyopic eye.

This test is also relatively gross. Plotting the boundary between the seeing and the blind area is subject to many errors, such as faulty patient responses to denote the disappearance or reappearance of the target, fixational inaccuracies, and examiner inaccuracies in making plot marks. Another possible source of error is the assumption that the two eyes are anatomically symmetrical. If not, an unequal displacement of the blind spots does not necessarily indicate eccentric fixation.

AFTERIMAGE TRANSFER TEST

The afterimage transfer test was originated by Brock (1950) and is based on the *normal* corresponding relationship of the two foveae: that the central foveal areas have the same local sign or give rise to common visual direction. Hence, the central foveal areas have a common central location in the cyclopean eye and an image falling on one fovea will be directionalized to the same spatial location as an image falling on the other fovea.

A vertical afterimage created by a monocularly presented stimulus which brackets the central fovea will therefore be projected into space so that it appears to bracket the image falling on the fovea of the other eye, when that eye fixates monocularly. This affords a means of identifying the image falling on the central fovea of one eye by determining which of a series of targets on a scale appears to be bracketed by the vertical afterimage originating from the other, now occluded, eye. By knowing which of the targets has its image on the central fovea of the fixating eye, it is possible to ascertain whether fixation is centric or eccentric. If fixation is centric, the vertical afterimage will be observed to bracket the fixation target as its image is falling on the foveal center of the fixating eye. If fixation is eccentric, the image of the fixation target is not stimulating the central fovea; the image of some other target on the scale is. The vertical afterimage now will be observed not about the fixation target but, instead, about the target which intercepts the visual axis and whose image is stimulating the central fovea.

Should a horizontal and vertical scale be presented with the fixation target at its center, the perceived location of the afterimage, in reference to the scale, will reveal the direction of the visual axis of the fixating eye and the location of the retinal area used for fixation.

In the testing procedure, Brock recommends that the vertical afterimage be created by a bright tubular light source whose center is shielded by an opaque band with a small central opening, the opening serving as a fixation target. The apparatus usually used for the Hering or Bielschowsky afterimage test may be used for this purpose. An adapted strobe light is preferred, however, as the afterimage may be instantaneously induced.

In unilateral amblyopia, the nonamblyopic eye fixates the dot light source, the other eye being occluded, and is exposed to the vertically oriented light filament situated approximately 4 feet from the eye (for approximately 20 seconds if a standard light filament is used). Following exposure and the creation of the vertical afterimage, the stimulated eye fixates the central zero mark on a scale calibrated for the distance of fixation, the amblyopic eye remaining occluded. Since it is assumed that the same retinal area is used for the fixation of the dot light source and the zero on the scale, the vertical afterimage should be seen about the zero fixation mark on the scale and the dot afterimage of the fixated light source should be seen centered in the zero.

This part of the procedure is for indoctrination—to provide some insight into the afterimage effect and its projected localization in reference to the fixation target. Following indoctrination, the non-amblyopic eye is again stimulated by the light filament to reinforce the afterimage. The occlusion is shifted to the nonamblyopic eye, and the amblyopic eye attempts to fixate the zero mark on the scale. The patient's task is to identify the location of the afterimage, induced in the now occluded nonamblyopic eye, as he fixates the central target on the scale with the amblyopic eye. Blinking the eyelids or flashing the room lights will assist in maintaining the afterimage effect.

Centric fixation is indicated if the vertical afterimage appears centered about the fixation target. In eccentric fixation, the afterimage will be observed to bracket vertically the target number whose image is stimulating the central fovea of the fixating amblyopic eye. For example, if a right amblyopic eye fixates eccentrically with an area 2 degrees nasal to the foveal center, the image of the target 2 degrees to the left of the fixation target will fall to the foveal center (as number 2 on a scale calibrated in degrees). Since the light stimulation to the nonamblyopic eye was directly above and below the foveal center and since number 2 on the scale is stimulating the foveal center of the amblyopic eye, the afterimage will appear to bracket number 2 to the left of the central fixation target. This indicates that the visual axis is not directed to the central fixation target but is deviated to its left by 2 degrees. The diagnosis would then be an eccentric fixation of a magnitude of 2 degrees, the site used being nasal to the fovea (since the afterimage was to the left of the fixation target).

Hauser and Burian (1957), in evaluating Brock's test, found that the results were influenced by the type of fixation target presented to the amblyopic eye. By reversing the test procedure (by providing an afterimage to the amblyopic eye and then having the normal eye fixate the central target of the scale), some patients who previously demonstrated eccentric fixation demonstrated normal fixation. They attributed the apparent switch to centric fixation to the more intensive fixation stimulus provided by the light filament compared to the weaker fixation stimulus of the zero on the target scale. To confirm their conclusion, they replaced the zero on the scale with a small light source and repeated the test in the routine manner (afterimage derived from normal eye). Some tendency was found to revert to centric fixation when the amblyopic eye fixated the light soure on the scale instead of the zero.

An obstacle to the use of the afterimage transfer test is that misleading conclusions may be reached if anomalous correspondence is present. The test is predicated on the fact that the fovea of each eye gives rise to common visual direction, that is, on normal correspondence; that the image stimulating the fovea of the amblyopic eye will be identified by the location of the afterimage derived from stimulation of the vertical retinal meridian of the other eye. Thus, even though the two eyes are stimulated separately, the end result is as though there were binocular stimulation, the *persistence* of stimulation of the normal eye being represented by the afterimage while the amblyopic eye is being stimulated.

Should anomalous correspondence be present, the foveal centers of the two eyes no longer give rise to a common visual direction. The fovea of one eye is associated directionally with some other retinal area (the anomalous associated area). Under such conditions, the image falling on the fovea of the amblyopic eye will not be identified by the perceived location of the afterimage. The afterimage will be perceived to bracket the number on the scale whose image is stimulating the anomalous, associated area in the amblyopic eye. This is so because this area, rather than the fovea of the amblyopic eye, is directionally associated with the fovea of the normal eye. In other words, the afterimage, instead of revealing whether or not fixation is eccentric, will be an indication of the angle of anomaly or the magnitude of the angular shift in common visual direction from the fovea to the anomalous, associated area.

To illustrate this point, assume a 10-degree right esotropia with anomalous correspondence and an angle of anomaly of 10 degrees. The straight-ahead visual direction normally possessed by the fovea of the right eye is therefore shifted 10 degrees to the nasal retina. If the afterimage transfer test is conducted in the usual manner and if fixation is centric, the afterimage, instead of being localized about the zero on the scale (as it would be in normal corespondence), is localized about the number 10 on the scale, to the right of the zero. That is, the image of number 10 is falling on the anomalous, associated area, and that is where the afterimage will be seen. If one is unaware of the existence of anomalous correspondence, this response would be construed to indicate eccentric fixation of a magnitude of 10 degrees.

Should a 2-degree nasal eccentric fixation be present in the same case, the afterimage will be seen about number 8 on the right side of the scale, although the image falling on the fovea is number 2 on the left side of the scale.

As a further illustration, if the same case had a 10-degree nasal eccentric fixation (the anomalous, associated area and the eccentric fixation site at the same retinal location), the afterimage would be seen about the zero on the scale because the image of the zero is falling on the anomalous, associated area.

Eccentric fixation may thus be diagnosed when none exists; if it does exist, its true extent may not be revealed and, under certain circumstances, it may go undetected even though it is large.

It is apparent that this test cannot be used if anomalous correspondence is present unless its diagnosis and measurement have already been made. For this reason one should rely on truly monocular tests —tests which do not depend on common visual direction—to detect eccentric fixation.

FUNDUS CAMERA

An ideal method not only of diagnosing fixation behavior but also of obtaining a permanent record of fixation response is a technique devised by von Noorden, Allen and Burian (1959). Into a Zeiss Nordenson fundus camera they incorporated a fixation target on a glass slide positioned between the ophthalmoscope and the camera lenses. The fixation target is a small black dot, 0.25 mm in diameter, centered in a 2-mm circle. As with the Visuscope, the fixation dot casts a shadow on the fundus, its fundus location revealing the retinal site used for fixation (See Figure 14 in Chapter 17). Photographs made for a series of fixations provide the basis for a precise diagnosis and allow comparisons with fixation responses after training.

Steady Fixation

In attempting to fixate a stationary target monocularly, an amblyopic eye, particularly one with strabismic amblyopia, frequently demonstrates an unsteadiness which may range from a mild exaggeration of the normal micromovements to an easily observed searching or nystagmoid type of movement. The degree of instability of fixation generally varies with the type of fixation (centric or eccentric), the consistency in location of the site used for fixation, and the extent of reduction in visual acuity. Typically, the unsteadiness is more marked when fixation is eccentric, when the site used for fixation is variable, and when visual acuity is markedly reduced. The steadiness of fixation therefore should be noted during the diagnostic workup by carefully observing the amblyopic eye as it attempts to fixate a stationary target monocularly at both far and near distances. Such observations may be made simultaneously while conducting other tests, such as those for visual acuity or eccentric fixation.

Pursuit and Saccadic Fixation

As in steady fixation, the ability of an amblyopic eye to continuously fixate a moving target or to shift fixation abruptly from one target to another is frequently found to be poor. Pursuit and saccadic fixation demands are more difficult than those of steady fixation, and irregularities present on steady fixation may be accentuated when pursuit or saccadic movements are attempted.

In pursuit demands, instead of a smooth rotational movement at a speed and path corresponding to that of the target, the movement is often jerky, nystagmoid, lagging behind the demand and not corresponding to the path followed by the target. In saccadic demands, instead of a swift and accurate movement to the second target, the eye may demonstrate a slowness of response and searching or corrective movements before finally assuming fixation of the second target.

Pursuit movements may be tested by means of a manually controlled target. A penlight may be used, or the Branchaud Wand, which has the added feature of a flickering light source, the flickering only apparent when fixation is not foveal. A number of motor-driven rotating fixation targets may also be used for this purpose, such as the Keystone Rotator, which has a strobe light attachment which flickers only if it is fixated inaccurately. Since target speed affects performance, the test should start with a slow movement.

A saccadic fixation demand may be presented by two hand-held targets, by directing fixation in turn to strategically placed distant targets or targets presented by means of a stereoscope, or by photographing with an Ophthalmograph or a Reading Eye the path the eye follows in fixating a series of closely spaced targets.

CHAPTER 13

Tests of
Spatial Localization

Anomalous spatial location is a frequent accompaniment of eccentric fixation. When an eccentric fixator attempts to localize a target which is monocularly fixated by the amblyopic eye, and when no clues or opportunities are afforded for corrective movements, the subjective localization of the target typically is not in agreement with its true physical location.

The presence of anomalous spatial localization tends to indicate that the principal visual direction is not associated with the eccentric retinal site which possesses the retinomotor value of zero, that incorrect or inaccurate information is received concerning the movement and positioning of the eye on fixating, or that localization of objects in space in reference to the self is vague and ill-defined.

If the straight-ahead direction and the retinomotor value of zero are both associated with the same eccentric site, one would expect spatial localization to be correct, just as in normal fixation in which the central fovea possesses both the straight-ahead direction and the retinomotor value of zero. If the principal visual direction remains associated with the foveal center while the retinomotor value of zero is located elsewhere, or if the motor information is incorrect, a conflict of localization cues results.

Past pointing serves as an analogy for this conflict. In past pointing, the eye rotates in the field of action of a recently paretic extraocular muscle in an attempt to fixate a gross target. Apparently, the impression is gained that the eye has rotated the required amount although, due to restricted motility, it has rotated insufficiently. Localization of the target is as though the eye rotated the correct amount and the target's image is stimulating an off-center retinal site with the visual axis correctly positioned. For example, if the right eye lags on attempting to fixate a target to the right, the image of the target will fall to the nasal side of the foveal center. The resulting localization of the nasal image appears to be from a reference position as if the eye rotated the correct amount; that the visual axis is directed to the location of the target, but that the target's image is still at its same nasal location. The image is therefore localized farther in the direction of the displacement of the target, or past the target, by an angle equal to the lag by which the eye misses foveal fixation.

A similar localization phenomenon appears to occur in functional eccentric fixation, although the nature of the localization error has not yet been experimentally determined.

Von Noorden has attempted to differentiate eccentric fixation on the basis of whether the patient feels that fixation is with the eye directed straight to the target (true eccentric fixation) or to the side of it (eccentric viewing). The feeling that the eye is directed straight to the target indicates, according to von Noorden, that the straight-ahead direction has shifted from the foveal center to the eccentric site.

Caution should be exercised in making this assumption solely on the basis of the patient's subjective assessment of how his eye is aimed. It is quite likely that the patient is not capable of precise awareness of the alignment of his eye with respect to the target, or of the target's location relative to himself, as would a patient with normal foveal fixation, with peak visual acuity at the foveal center and with a sensitive discrimination of direction. This is evidenced by the fact that anomalous spatial localization is present in eccentric fixators who judge the eye to be directed straight to the target.

An explanation by Brock (1967) for anomalous spatial localization does not involve either the zero retinomotor value or the principal visual direction of the amblyopic eye, but rather cyclopean projection. He states that localization in amblyopia is anomalous because the fixation target is localized in space as though its image were stimulating the corresponding area of the occluded eye. Localization is as if the occluded eye were fixating in the direction it is turned behind the occluder.

If this concept is correct and if a large-angle strabismus is present, the perceptual localization of the target would be displaced from the true physical location by an angular amount approximately equal to the strabismic deviation. Ordinarily, this does not occur. The perceptual error in localization is usually relatively small and does not appear to be equal to, or correlated with, the angle of strabismus.

Spatial localization tests may be performed on any of a variety of instruments, but a demand common to most is the localization of a fixated target with a hand-held pointer, usually shielded from view.

GROSS EVALUATION

Spatial localization may be grossly examined by having the patient point to, or touch, a monocularly fixated target such as the light source of a penlight, a target on a near-point acuity chart, or the fixation target when checking for eccentric fixation with the Maxwell's spot or the Haidinger's brush technique. Errors in spatial judgment will be revealed by a consistent failure to locate the target correctly. Gross evaluations may also be made by noting the path of the patient as he walks toward a monocularly fixated target.

In using such methods, one must be on the alert for the patient's compensation of his errors of judgment, which become obvious to him as the target is approached.

PROJECTIONOMETERS

A more sophisticated method for evaluating spatial localization is with the Landolt projectionometer. This instrument consists of a horizontally extending shelf fitted perpendicularly into a vertical shelf which contains a vertical fixation line just above and a tangent scale just below its junction with the horizontal shelf. The patient, with his head placed at eye level against the outer edge of the horizontal shelf, monocularly fixates the vertical line and indicates its perceived location by means of a hand-held pointer (or his finger) positioned below the horizontal shelf and thus shielded from view. The location of the pointer on the tangent scale below the shelf, in relation to the locus of the fixated vertical line above the shelf, will reveal whether spatial localization is correct or anomalous.

Another instrument for testing spatial localization is the Alabaster projectionometer. This device consists of a horizontal, semicircular platform containing at its circular periphery, on its upper side, a metal railing to support a movable light source controlled by the examiner and, on its lower side, a similar railing supporting a wooden ball controlled by the patient. The patient, with his head positioned at the midpoint of the flat side, monocularly fixates the light source and attempts to position the wooden ball beneath the shelf so that it is directly under the perceived location of the fixated light. With this instrument, one has the added advantage of testing spatial localization at any desired direction of gaze, not just the straight-ahead position.

MADDOX PROJECTION TEST

The Maddox Projection Test offers still another approach to the examination of spatial localization. It consists of a white card in the center of which is printed, on both sides and in the same location, a 1-inch-long black vertical line. The card is held directly in front of one eye at a near distance of approximately 6 inches. The patient monocularly fixates the line, the other eye being occluded, and indicates its apparent location by reaching around and pointing on the back of the card. The pointer is thus shielded from view and, since an identically located line is on the reverse side, the examiner can ascertain whether localization is correct or anomalous.

SMITH PROJECTION PLATE

William S. Smith (1950) has devised a projection plate which is useful in both the testing and the training of spatial localization. The plate contains a number of colored drawings of familiar objects, the outline and interior of which contain a number of small holes (Figure 13). The test is performed at a near distance and at eye level. The patient monocularly fixates a hole selected by the examiner and attempts to place a colored toothpick directly into this hole. The patient holds the toothpick in front of and close to the fixating eye, aims it at the hole, and then moves it swiftly toward the hole.

Since the pointer and its target are both visible, the movement must be constant and rapid. This will tend to prevent corrective move-

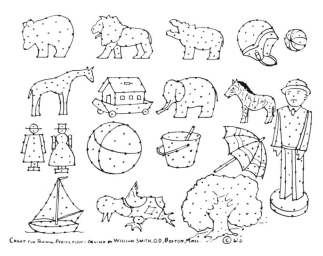

Figure 13. Smith's Projection Plate. (*From Smith:* Clinical Orthoptic Procedure, *2nd ed., St. Louis, 1954, the C. V. Mosby Co.*)

ments, which otherwise would occur if anomalous localization is present, and the patient realizes as the pointer approaches the hole that it is going to miss. If a slow but constant movement of the toothpick is permitted, and if anomalous spatial localization is present, the corrective movement will be manifested by the path the toothpick takes to the hole. It will curve toward it just before striking it, much as if an attempt were made to perform this task through a displacing prism. If the movement is swift, the corrective movements will occur after the toothpick strikes the plate and misses the opening. A series of searching movements is made in an attempt to place the pick in the hole.

The tests described for spatial localization should be performed several times to determine whether or not an error is consistently made and, if so, whether the error is constant or variable. Some motor dexterity is necessarily involved, and small, random and inconstant errors are more likely to be due to motor control of the hand than to perceptual errors in spatial judgment.

Head posture may have a bearing on the results. If a head tilt or turn is present, spatial localization tests should be performed both with the head in its abnormal posture and then with the head positioned straight. Anomalous spatial localization may be manifested only when the test is performed with the head positioned straight, indicating an interplay between spatial localization and head orientation (Smith, 1950). As Duke-Elder pointed out (1949), visual direction is dependent upon an interplay and coordination between visual and postural reflexes. Proprioceptive impulses from the neck muscles and from the labyrinth in response to movements of the head or changes in body position, impulses from the extraocular muscles on movement of the eyes, and impulses from the retinal receptors are all considered to play a part in orienting the self in space and the directions of objects in reference to the eye and to the self.

If anomalous spatial localization is detected, its average extent and direction should be noted. Anomalous spatial localization strongly indicates eccentric fixation.

CHAPTER **14**

Tests of
Foveal Integrity

Central Relative Scotoma

In amblyopia ex anopsia, a functional, central, relative scotoma is frequently present, varying in size from approximately 1 to 6 degrees. Relative scotoma is the consequence of constant central suppression and is characterized by reduced sensitivity to form stimuli, by loss of precise directionalization, and by failure to perceive images of targets stimulating this area under binocular conditions (suppression).

Clinical approaches to detecting and measuring this relative scotoma do not attempt to plot, under monocular conditions, isopters of sensitivity to form or color stimuli or to local sign. They usually involve binocular conditions and plot areas of suppression within which target content has disappeared. The scotoma detected under the latter condition is thus relative to binocular stimulation, when central suppression is operative, and may not be found under monocular test conditions, when suppression is inoperative. It would therefore be more descriptive to refer to the scotoma detected in this manner as a *suppression scotoma* because its existence and size are dependent upon the area of the central field that is intensely suppressed.

Testing procedures designed to detect and measure a suppression area usually introduce a reduced environment characterized by limited fields of vision and simplified target content. Under such test conditions, the suppression responses present in the normal spatial environment tend to break down, and only the most intense, those at the fovea, persist. The size of the central area of the visual field of the amblyopic eye in which the target content has disappeared is thus smaller than the suppression scotoma present in the normal environment. If suppression is not intense, the scotoma may go undetected during testing, although it is present and operative in the normal environment.

Suppression scotoma detected under these reduced conditions is generally considered to be an indication of the size of the scotoma, which is relative to form vision or local sign. That is, the area intensely suppressed in the amblyopic eye is also the area which can be expected to demonstrate depressed sensitivity to form and local sign. But that is not always the case because suppression scotoma can also occur in strabismus without associated amblyopia (as in alternating strabismus).

The complete disappearance of target content manifested under binocular conditions also may be due to an organic defect and not suppression; that is, to absolute scotoma, not functional relative scotoma. A field study, therefore, should also include a test conducted under monocular conditions. Central scotoma found during monocular testing indicates a blind area due to organic causes, not to suppression or to the effect of suppression.

The detection of an absolute central scotoma indicates that the amblyopia is organic in nature, or that it has an organic component, and that visual acuity can be no better than that provided by the retinal area surrounding the absolute scotoma.

Tests for Central Scotoma

The patient may reveal an absolute scotoma during monocular visual acuity testing by a comment that the target, or parts of it, disappear when he directs his eye straight to it and that in order to see the target he must direct his eye to the side of it. This response should not be confused with improved acuity for targets to the side of the one fixated. In such an instance, the fixated target is visible and the improved acuity may be attributed to eccentric fixation, the image of the target adjacent to the fixated target stimulating the more central retina, which is capable of superior acuity.

An absolute central scotoma may be detected and measured with customary field plotting equipment, such as a tangent screen or stereocampimeter. Monocular procedures are preferred, so as not to incorrectly diagnose a suppression scotoma for an absolute scotoma. Testing may be performed monocularly, provided the amblyopic eye has steady fixation. The fixation target should be as small as possible to assist in stabilizing fixation, and the plotting target should be 0.5 degree or less to make possible the detection of small central scotomata.

Central field investigation is often more difficult to perform monocularly, with the amblyopic eye fixating. The fixation target may tend to disappear and fixation control may be extremely poor, even if the target remains visible. An erratically fixating eye prevents detection of a small central scotoma in its visual field.

Fixation controls commonly used on a tangent screen, if an absolute central scotoma is present, are circles of varying diameter or white line marks (vertical, above and below, horizontal to the sides) centered about the fixation target. The eye is directed to the apparent center of the circle target or to the apparent crossing point of the line marks.

VISUSCOPE AND PROJECTOSCOPE

An absolute central scotoma may be detected with the Visuscope (21) or the Projectoscope (11). The patient directs the amblyopic eye straight ahead (not at the star target), the other eye being occluded, while the examiner centers the shadow over the foveolar reflex. Failure to perceive the star pattern indicates central scotoma. Its extent may be approximated by moving the shadow in various directions until it becomes visible.

STEREOCAMPIMETRY

The stereocampimeter provides a means of investigating the central field of the amblyopic eye while fixation is maintained by the fellow eye. This, of course, introduces a binocular situation and the possibility that central suppression will cause the plotting target to disappear. Should fixation be highly erratic, however, a binocular approach is necessary to render the eyes motionless during the field investigation.

In utilizing a binocular arrangement, the type of retinal correspondence, the magnitude of strabismic deviation and the target content should be considered. Retinal correspondence becomes important, for now it is necessary to locate the region in the field of vision of the nonfixating amblyopic eye which corresponds to central vision. In strabismus with normal correspondence, the central field is localized by determining the locus in the field where the plotting target is directionalized to the same locos as is the fixation target is directed. For example, if a small circular fixation target is used, the location of the intersection of the visual axis of the amblyopic eye with the plane of the plotting field is indicated by the locus where the plotting target appears centered in the circular fixation target, or would be centered if the plotting target disappears as the image of the fixation target is approached.

That no longer holds in anomalous correspondence because the foveae do not possess the attribute of common visual direction. Under such circumstances, before field plotting is attempted it is necessary to determine the objective angle of strabismus with an instrument having essentially the same focal length as the stereocampimeter— an instrument such as the Troposcope. An allowance is then made on the stereocampimeter for this deviation. Thus, if the objective angle is 10 degrees of esotropia and if the right eye is amblyopic, the approximate location of the intersection of the visual axis of the right amblyopic eye with the plane of the plotting field will be 10 degrees to the left of the zero or "ortho" position.

Whether correspondence is normal or anomalous, it may be necessary to use auxiliary prisms to align the central field of vision of the eye in the center of the field of view of the instrument. Otherwise, the central field of vision may be to the side, or even out of the plotting field, depending on the magnitude of the strabismic deviation.

The charts used with the stereocampimeter contain a scaled grid pattern, and the fixation targets presented to the two eyes are at the center of radially intersecting lines. Normally, the grid patterns and the pattern surrounding the fixation targets are to be fused. In strabismus, however, fusion is usually absent and plotting is simplified by using the reverse side of the chart, presenting a plain black field to the amblyopic eye and a small white fixation target to the fixating eye. The confusion and rivalry of the lines are thus eliminated and more valid findings are obtained.

The procedure for investigating the central field is accomplished in the routine manner, taking care that fixation is constantly maintained, that the eyes remain motionless, and that the plotting target is 0.5 degree or less.

STEREOGRAMS

One of the most common clinical means of detecting a suppression scotoma is to present superimposition or fusion targets by means of a stereoscope, vectograms, anaglyphs or Polaroid filters and to note whether or not any of the target content disappears. The maximum size target which disappears, or the horizontal and vertical range through which it is not seen, serves as an indication of the size of the suppression scotoma. The disappearance of a target under such conditions, however, occurs in any suppressing strabismic, whether or not amblyopia is present, and thus its manifestation does not necessarily correspond to an area of depressed sensitivity in an amblyopic eye. Again, the type of retinal correspondence must be known in order to properly identify the region of the retina which is suppressed.

BROCK PROJECTION BOX

The Brock Projection Box (Brock and Schechter, 1942; Brock, 1943, 1951) is an instrument specifically designed to detect a central scotoma. It consists of a small housing containing a vertically orientated light source beneath which is situated a target composed of a 2-degree red circle with a black dot at its center. The transilluminated image of the target is reflected by a 45-degree inclined front surface mirror through a collimating lens and peephole.

The device is fixed before the normal eye by means of an attached headband so that the peephole is directly in front of the normal eye and fixation is directed to the black dot. A second device housing a bright light source and fitted with an adjustable diaphragm providing an aperture opening ranging in size from 1 mm to 5 mm is placed in front of the patient, in a completely dark room, at a distance of from 6 inches to 6 feet, depending on the severity of the amblyopia. With fixation constantly maintained on the black dot, the patient is instructed to move his head in the appropriate direction until the non-fixated light source, visible only to the amblyopic eye, appears directly beneath the red circle. Then he adjusts his head so that the fixated target appears to move downward over the light source. A central scotoma is suggested if the light scource consistently disappears when superimposition of the light and the black dot is attempted, or if a corona of light is seen surrounding the black fixation dot. To avoid retinal adaptation and disappearance of the light for this reason, superimposition of the light source and the target should not be maintained once it is experienced.

To verify the presence of central scotoma, the test may be repeated with the Projection Box in front of the amblyopic eye and the light source fixated by the normal eye, central scotoma being confirmed if the black dot disappears as it approaches superimposition on the fixated light source.

This test can only be performed when normal correspondence is present because it is dependent on the foveae giving rise to common visual direction. Caution must be exercised in interpreting results; the disappearance of a target on attempted superimposition may be due not only to an absolute central scotoma but also to central suppression, retinal rivalry or retinal adaptation. Hence, if a scotoma is found, it is advisable to confirm the finding by other tests.

POSTURE BOARD

Another device devised by Brock to investigate foveal integrity, but confined to cases of unilateral amblyopia without strabismus, is the Posture Board (15), a table-mounted, rectangular-shaped instrument composed of an 8½ x 11 inch sheet of red plastic elevated above a base plate by four corner supports. The red plastic sheet is fitted with four clips to hold targets placed over it. A hand-held rod containing a small white light source is positioned between the red plastic sheet and its supporting base so that the light is directed through the red plastic sheet and appears deep red. The chart used for this purpose (Retinal Integrity Test No. 1) consists of a grid with two small concentric circles at its center. The circles enclose five 20/20 reduced Snellen letters, one at the center of the inner circle and four in square formation in the outer circle. All marks are red on a white background.

Wearing any necessary lens correction, the patient views this target, positioned horizontally at a 16-inch distance, in a well-illuminated room and through complementary colored red and green filters, red in front of the amblyopic eye. Under these conditions, the red target content is not visible to the amblyopic eye, blending in with the red created by the red filter, but is visible to the other eye, appearing black through the green filter. The location of the central field of the amblyopic eye, which is determined earlier with a similarly constructed target (Binocular Posture Test No. 3), is marked lightly on the form with a red pencil (Eberhard Faber OKAY 636).

The patient is instructed to fixate carefully and continuously the central letter, visible only to the nonamblyopic eye, while the red light, visible only to the amblyopic eye, is moved toward it. Actually, the red light is moved toward the indicated location of the central field of the amblyopic eye, for in normal binocular functioning, when positioned on the visual axis of the amblyopic eye, it will be perceived as superimposed on the fixated letter. If an absolute or a suppression central scotoma is present, the red light will disappear as it approaches the scotomatous area, and the extent of the scotoma may then be plotted.

A shift in fixation by the nonamblyopic eye may occur to avoid the image of the red light from falling on the scotomatous region; this is indicated by a loss of definition of the fixation target when superimposed on by the red light.

RETINAL SENSITIVITY

Since the central relative scotoma in amblyopia ex anopsia is an area of decreased sensitivity, especially to form and local sign as manifested under monocular conditions, tests to evaluate central functioning should more properly be directed to the determination of isopters of relative sensitivity to form stimuli and local sign differentiation rather than to the detection and measurement of a suppression scotoma: that is, to changes, or lack of changes, in perception of stimuli rather than to the disappearance of stimuli. Clinically, that is usually not attempted because of the difficulty in performing such tests. They require maximum cooperation and fixation control and skilled observation, and even then the procedure is lengthy and fatiguing. Unfortunately, most patients on whom such an examination would be conducted are very young and accordingly show poor cooperation, fixation control and observations and are unable to perform consistently for even short periods of time.

Should a patient be able to meet these demands, isopters of relative sensitivity to form stimuli may be plotted by positioning a form stimulus, such as one or more rotatable Snellen Es of various known visual angles, along the arm of an arc perimeter, beginning at the periphery and progressing toward the straight-ahead monocularly fixated target. Identification of the form target for the tested retinal locations will determine if the central vision demonstrates poorer acuity than the more peripheral vision.

The difficulty in conducting this test is that the area expected to demonstrate reduced sensitivity is small, encompassing a few degrees or less to each side of the fixation target, and the temptation to shift fixation to the plotting target is almost too great to resist. In addition, the test requires the introduction of progressively smaller targets, each of which is introduced from at least four starting points, superior and inferior in the 90-degree meridian and nasal and temporal in the 180-degree meridian.

The tachistoscope may also be used for this purpose by flashing onto a screen form targets of known visual angles and known angular displacements from the fixation target. This method does simplify the fixation demand because the target is flashed at a speed in excess of one tenth of a second, eliminating the possibility of a shift in fixation.

In either of these two techniques, the type of fixation must be determined beforehand to relate the acuity findings to the correct retinal location.

IRVINE PRISM DISPLACEMENT TEST

Impairment of local sign in central vision may be examined by the Irvine Prism Displacement Test. Fixation is maintained on the central target of a tangent screen, or any other suitable target, the other eye being occluded, while a prism with its base-apex line in a given meridian is abruptly introduced in front of the fixating eye. The least amount of prism power which causes a just noticeable shift in the direction of the fixation target is taken as a measure of the limit of the relative scotoma for this meridian and for the direction of displacement of the retinal image. The procedure is repeated with the base-apex line in different meridians, and with the base in the opposite direction in the same meridian, until the boundaries of the relative scotoma have been ascertained. Fixation must be steady, the type of fixation must be known, and the existence of absolute central scotoma must be ruled out (otherwise this procedure will serve as a measurement of the absolute scotoma).

Color Vision

Color vision thresholds for various wavelengths of light may be higher in amblyopia ex anopsia, but it is generally believed that color vision is essentially normal. Color vision tests, therefore, are administered primarily for the purpose of differentiating between congenital amblyopia, or organic amblyopia, and functional amblyopia.

Congenital color vision defects are almost always bilateral. Thus, if an equal acuity reduction exists in the two eyes associated with a bilateral color vision anomaly, a hereditary and organic etiology is indicated and acuity training would not be productive. If acuity is reduced in both eyes but significantly better in one eye and if a bilateral color vision defect is present, an organic component is indicated and the acuity in the poorer eye, after corrective procedures, cannot be expected to improve beyond that of the better eye.

Unilateral amblyopia associated with deficient color perception only in the amblyopic eye may indicate a relative scotoma, much the same as for form vision, or of eccentric fixation and would not carry the same poor prognosis as a bilateral color vision defect.

Miscellaneous Considerations

Other clinical indications of a defect in foveal integrity include the failure to perceive the Haidinger's brushes or the Maxwell's spot and significant reduction in visual acuity in the neutral-density filter test.

The Hall Selection Test is frequently mentioned as a means of differentiating between amblyopia ex anopsia and congenital amblyopia, although it is of doubtful validity. Two red circular targets, 5 mm in diameter on a black background and 1½ inches apart, are presented to the amblyopic eye at a distance of 40 cm, the other eye being occluded. The patient fixates one disk and compares the relative brightness of the two disks (assuming the image of the fixated disk is falling on the fovea). A report of equal brightness of the fixated and the nonfixated disk is said to indicate congenital amblyopia and a poor prognosis. A report of greater brightness of the peripheral target is said to indicate amblyopia ex anopsia, the fixated target being dimmer as a result of a relative central scotoma.

Peripheral Visual Fields

A field study should be made, where possible, to examine the integrity and limits of the peripheral fields. This ensures that no pathological defect has been overlooked and, in suspect cases, serves as a check for hysterical amblyopia and the presence of tubular or spiral fields. Since amblyopia ex anopsia is an affliction of central vision, the peripheral fields in this condition should be intact and of normal limits. The blind spots of Mariotte of the two eyes, however, may be unequally displaced from the fixation target if a large angle of eccentric fixation is present in the amblyopic eye.

CHAPTER 15

The Prognosis

Prospects for the improvement or recovery of visual acuity depend primarily on the type of amblyopia, its duration and the age of onset, the type of treatment, and the patient's cooperation.

Of the organic types, prognosis is good in nutritional and tobacco amblyopia if duration is short and treatment is prompt; it varies considerably in toxic amblyopia, depending upon the toxic agent, but generally is poor; and it is poor in congenital amblyopia, although vision may spontaneously improve with the attainment of maximum development.

Of the functional types, prognosis is good in hysterical amblyopia with successful psychotherapy; it is poor in light deprivation amblyopia, unless treated very early in life; and is good in isoametropic amblyopia, provided the visual pathway is normal and corrective lenses are prescribed early in life. In amblyopia ex anopsia, prognosis depends upon many related factors. In anisometropic amblyopia, the prospect is good if the refractive error is corrected at an early age (before the age of 6) and if training is concurrently provided to aid in the recovery and development of vision. Similarly, in strabismic amblyopia prospects are good if treatment is started at an early age, regardless of whether fixation is centric or eccentric.

Prognosis becomes progressively poorer as treatment is delayed beyond the age of 5 or 6, both in anisometropic and in strabismic amblyopia, especially if onset is at birth or in infancy. Acuity improvement is more slowly attained, and hopes of achieving normal and complete development, with 20/20 vision, become progressively reduced with advancing age. Improvement in acuity is possible, however, even in adult life. A prolonged delay in initiating treatment does not necessarily preclude improvement, but it does reduce the degree of potential improvement and increases the time and effort required to accomplish the limited increase.

With delay in detection and treatment the chances for acuity improvement and its permanence become more dependent upon the coexistence of other anomalous visual habits.

Should eccentric fixation be present, the possibility of restoring centric fixation varies with its magnitude and variability. Larger, variable angles of eccentric fixation offer a better prognosis. The most difficult variety to break down is one in which fixation is steady and in which the retinal area employed for fixation is close to the foveal center and is consistently used. In this type, the eccentric fixation response is firmly established and, being close to the foveal center, is difficult to correct. Often, training may succeed in altering a large and variable angle of eccentric fixation to a stable small angle, with no further improvement possible. Even the best training techniques appear inadequate in providing an effective stimulus to encourage the small eye movement necessary to convert a small-angle eccentric fixation to centric fixation.

Delay in the treatment of strabismic amblyopia influences not only the speed and degree of acuity improvement but also its permanence. For acuity improvement to be sustained, normal binocular functioning must be established; that is, binocular fixation and central sensory fusion must occur. The longer the strabismus is present, the more resistant to treatment are such anomalous visual habits as suppression and anomalous correspondence, and the less is the likelihood of eliminating the strabismus. Without elimination of the strabismus, the causative factors of strabismic amblyopia continue to operate and a partial or complete loss of acuity improvement may be anticipated unless the strabismus has been changed to the alternating type.

Effective training procedures and patient (and parent) cooperation are vital components in predicting success in the treatment of amblyopia ex anopsia. A training program must be in earnest, with controlled stimulation maximally provided to the amblyopic eye. Intensive training, correctly applied and carried out, will produce acuity and fixation improvement to full potential in the shortest period of time. Haphazard training programs or failure to follow instructions faithfully will result in failure.

To determine the prognosis, it is important to diagnose the type of amblyopia. Congenital amblyopia is identified least clearly, especially if unilateral, and a definite differential diagnosis between congenital amblyopia and amblyopia ex anopsia may not be possible. If properly performed training fails to produce an improvement after four to six weeks, the condition can be considered congenital.

PART IV

Training Procedures

CHAPTER 16

Preliminary Considerations

The type of amblyopia that is most responsive to visual training is amblyopia ex anopsia. Training may also be beneficial in hastening an acuity improvement and in attaining maximum potential vision, after corrective lenses are provided, in isoametropic amblyopia.

It should be stressed that amblyopia ex anopsia is a preventable or easily reversible visual loss if its causes, unilateral strabismus and uncorrected anisometropia, are detected and receive attention early in life. Emphasis in clinical practice should therefore be concentrated on educating parents about the importance of routine visual examinations for preschool children and on instituting immediate preventive or remedial measures if a condition is found which could lead to, or already has caused, amblyopia ex anopsia. Prompt early treatment will eliminate or prevent the onset of amblyopia ex anopsia and the accompanying complication of eccentric fixation. It will also ensure normal and complete development of visual acuity and prevent the establishment or intensification of binocular adaptive anomalies such as suppression or anomalous correspondence.

REFRACTION AND PRESCRIBING

Refractive analysis has not been emphasized in this text; it is assumed that it will be performed in the customary manner, in accordance with the patient's age and cooperation. The subject is introduced not to elaborate on refractive techniques but to stress (1) the importance of performing a careful refraction to render maximum retinal focus, (2) the importance of prescribing corrective lenses *prior* to treatment even though the refractive error may be small, and (3) the need to repeat refractions as vision and responses improve either spontaneously from the wearing of lenses alone, as frequently occurs in refractive amblyopia, or as a result of vision training. Findings on reexamination often differ from the original, and changes in the correction are necessary to attain maximum vision.

From the standpoint of preventive care, it is most important to correct significant refractive errors immediately to provide the two eyes with sharply focused retinal images, normal and equal demands on accommodation, and normal demands on convergence. This does not necessarily imply the prescription of full corrections for the complete neutralization of ametropia, for it may be desirable to depart from the full prescription.

The correction of significant refractive errors during the first few years of life may prevent unilateral esotropia and the consequent amblyopia in hypermetropes with high ACA ratios. Anisometropes would have no need to suppress a more blurred retinal image, a reaction which not only leads to amblyopia but also may lead to strabismus. Should a constant unilateral strabismus already be present, other preventive steps must be taken in addition to the prescription of corrective lenses to ensure normal development of fixation and visual acuity and to prevent binocular anomalies.

A consideration in prescribing for anisometropia is the possibility of aniseikonia. Generally, differences in the spherical component of the refractive errors are primarily axial in nature, while differences in the cylindrical component are refractive in nature. Hence, aniseikonia resulting from the prescription of refractive corrections for even highly unequal spherical refractive errors may not seriously impede sensory fusion. The lateral, and especially vertical, prism effects induced when the lines of sight leave the optical centers of the lenses, however, may create a motor fusion problem. This is one reason why contact lenses may prove superior to spectacles for the correction of higher anisometropic refractive errors, even though aniseikonia may result.

It is usually not possible to measure aniseikonic errors when prescribing spectacle lens corrections for anisometropic patients of preschool age. Thus the selection of front surface curvatures and center thicknesses to minimize aniseikonia is based on mathematical computation, keeping in mind what is optically and cosmetically practical and remembering that differences in the spherical component are usually primarily axial in origin.

If amblyopia ex anopsia is present, significant refractive errors should be corrected before training begins. Training to improve fixation and visual acuity should be performed under the most favorable conditions; an essential prerequisite is to provide a sharply focused image. As mentioned, this alone might result in improved vision in anisometropia and high isoametropia, if unaccompanied by strabismus.

TRAINING OBJECTIVES

The aim of visual training for amblyopia ex anopsia is to establish steady centric fixation, normal directional values, and maximum and peak visual acuity at the central fovea. If this is accomplished, the foveal center will possess the zero retinomotor value and the straight-ahead (principal) visual direction, and the visual pathway of the affected eye will be in normal operation, free from inhibition or suppression influences or their residual effects.

To achieve these objectives fully and quickly, the amblyopic eye is exposed to controlled stimulation which is intensive, repetitive and specifically designed to eliminate malfunctioning and to promote normal functioning.

It should be remembered that in strabismic amblyopia training to attain normal fixation and maximum acuity is but the initial phase of a training program whose ultimate objective is to establish normal sensory and motor fusion. If this goal is not attained and if the strabismic condition persists, deterioration of fixation and acuity improvements can be anticipated.

CHAPTER 17

Occlusion

Occlusion of the sound eye for the treatment of amblyopia ex anopsia is one of the earliest forms of visual training. It was advocated as early as 1743 by du Buffon to stimulate the deviated amblyopic eye in strabismus. It remains the most commonly used initial step to establish normal fixation reflex and to restore normal vision through forced fixation and forced cortical reception and utilization of impulses from the amblyopic eye. It also serves to break down suppression and anomalous retinal correspondence by preventing their continued use.

In very young patients with unilateral strabismus of recent onset, occlusion serves to prevent these conditions from occurring by promoting the continued use of the fixation reflex and the continued development of visual acuity.

Inverse Occlusion

Until recent years, the nonamblyopic eye routinely received occlusion. With greater knowledge of eccentric fixation and of clinical techniques for its detection, measurement and treatment came fears that occlusion practiced in this manner would intensify eccentric fixation if it was present would intensify anomalous fixation. Bangerter (1953) thus advocated for strabismic amblyopia with eccentric fixation total and constant occlusion of the amblyopic eye for a period of from one to two months prior to training and then between training sessions, a technique known as inverse occlusion. Such occlusion is continued until fixation becomes either unsteady centric or steady centric; then the standard approach to occlusion is practiced, the unaffected eye being occluded. The reasons given for occluding the amblyopic eye are to weaken, through disuse, the eccentric fixation and to remove the influences of suppression and anomalous correspondence.

ANALYSIS

Although there was little experimental evidence to sustain the premise that occlusion of the sound eye would intensify or strengthen an existing eccentric fixation, regardless of its characteristics, inverse occlusion quickly became the popular method for handling eccentric fixation. This repudiation of the standard approach of occluding the normal eye deserved more careful thought, since up to that time standard occlusion, when properly practiced and combined with visual training, had generally proven effective in improving both acuity and fixation.

One reason given for occluding the amblyopic eye in strabismus is to prevent continued use of eccentric fixation. Only infrequently, however, does the image of the fixation object stimulate the same area of the retina in the deviating eye under binocular conditions that is used for fixation under monocular conditions. This is immediately apparent when the fixating eye is covered and the deviating eye is observed to move to assume fixation. In unilateral strabismus, the amblyopic eye does not fixate actively (eccentrically). Rather, it deviates away from fixation and assumes a passive role, its movements controlled by movements of the fixating eye and its posture primarily one of subserving acquired suppression relationships. Thus if eccentric fixation is not operative under binocular conditions, as is the rule, the occlusion of the amblyopic eye for the purpose of promoting disuse of eccentric fixation serves no real purpose. It is in disuse, whether the amblyopic eye is occluded or not. If this were the only reason for occluding the amblyopic eye, neither eye would need to be occluded.

A second reason given for occluding the amblyopic eye is to eliminate the influences of suppression and anomalous correspondence. These two binocular anomalies could affect the fixation response of the amblyopic eye, as has been discussed under theories of eccentric fixation. The same can be claimed, however, for occlusion of the nonamblyopic eye.

Another factor pertinent to inverse occlusion is the patient's age. If conventional occlusion of the normal eye begins early in life (before the age of 4), assuming a healthy eye, almost invariably fixation improves and vision quickly returns to that expected for the age level. Thus at early ages inverse occlusion may be contraindicated.

A further consideration concerns the characteristics of eccentric fixation. The greater the unsteadiness and the larger and more variable the angle, the less likely will eccentric fixation be intensified if the sound eye is occluded. But a site of fixation which is close to the foveal center and which is steadily and constantly employed may become intensified if the nonamblyopic eye is occluded. This latter type, therefore, may be more suitably treated with inverse occlusion than with standard occlusion.

TRAINING REQUIREMENTS

The passive nature of inverse occlusion bears importantly on training requirements. In conventional occlusion, as stated, the purpose is to promote increased stimulation to the amblyopic eye and to force cortical reception and interpretation of the central impulses from the eye, and so in time to attain improvement in fixation and visual acuity. In inverse occlusion, the amblyopic eye is deprived of all stimulation except during training. Since improvement in fixation and acuity is ultimately dependent upon controlled stimulation to the amblyopic eye, not upon deprivation of stimulation, the time devoted to training becomes especially critical if inverse occlusion is employed.

In treating amblyopia ex anopsia, Bangerter either confines his patients to a hospital especially staffed and equipped for visual training or requires that they attend "school" daily at this hospital. The patients are thus exposed to expertly conducted training which is administered for at least 2 hours a day and carried on for up to approximately 4 weeks.

Training carried out in this manner is undoubtedly one of the primary reasons for reported successes with inverse occlusion. Concentrated training provided daily by skilled persons utilizing specialized instrumentation affords sufficient stimulation to the amblyopic eye to permit its occlusion between training periods. If that cannot be done, it would appear that standard occlusion would be more effective.

Ideally, regardless of the occlusion, training approach or type of training problem, the more time that is devoted to effective training per day, the greater and faster will be the improvement. Concentrated and intensive training, therefore, is highly desirable and, in stubborn problems, may make the difference between success and failure. In amblyopia ex anopsia, if patients can be trained several hours every day, it is probable that no occlusion is necessary whether fixation is centric or eccentric.

Although there have been attempts to imitate the Bangerter "amblyopa school" (a summer camp sponsored by the Beale Eye Foundation in San Francisco is one example), supervised training, at least in the United States, is typically given only two or three times a week and then for only half or three quarters of an hour. Such brief and sporadic training is inadequate when practicing inverse occlusion, just as occlusion of the normal eye would be if it were practiced for only a few hours a day, a few times a week.

REEVALUATION

Sometime after the introduction of the inverse occlusion technique, several reports both evaluated this approach and reevaluated the standard occlusion approach. Urist (1955) used conventional occlusion in treating patients whose angle of eccentric fixation equaled strabismic deviation and found that, when 20/200 or better could be achieved, all patients developed centric fixation, with those of preschool age showing the most improvement in vision.

Burian (1956) challenged the concept that occlusion of the fixating eye reinforces eccentric fixation, reporting success with total standard occlusion regardless of the type of fixation, especially in young subjects. He did find, however, that with eccentric fixation the treatment was more prolonged and the improvement tended to be more unstable.

Viefhues (1957) found that occlusion of the nonamblyopic eye of infants would in itself quickly restore centric fixation, and he recommended such occlusion whether fixation was centric or eccentric. In applying early constant occlusion to the sound eye in strabismic amblyopia with eccentric fixation, Scully (1961) reported that all but 1 out of 57 patients reverted to centric fixation. Barnard (1962) found conventional occlusion effective in patients under age 6 even though eccentric fixation was present, although he had better success when it was preceded by several months of inverse occlusion. Inverse occlusion combined with training was found most effective for patients with onset between the ages of 1 and 3 whose present age was from 6 to 10. Similar results were obtained with conventional occlusion in patients up to the age of 5 by Steer (1964), who preferred conventional occlusion alone, particularly for those under age 3. He recommended inverse occlusion interrupted by periods of standard occlusion for children from 3 to 5, especially if fixation was steady eccentric.

Von Noorden (1965) found no evidence that conventional occlusion reinforced anomalous fixation; rather, it proved superior to inverse occlusion for both fixation and acuity in children up to age 4. Von Noorden felt that inverse occlusion might be of use in older children who failed to improve with conventional occlusion. Parks and Friendly (1966) agree with von Noorden. They performed constant occlusion of the fixating eye in children under 4 years of age with gross eccentric fixation, and relatively quickly obtained centric fixation in 116 out of 117 subjects, 86 percent achieving 20/30 vision or better as measured with the illiterate E. The occlusion period required to obtain centric fixation averaged 6 weeks if started by age 2, and 3 months if started between ages 2 and 4.

VerLee and Iacobucci (1967) compared two groups of 50 strabis- mic amblyopes, one group treated solely with total occlusion of the sound eye for an average of 3 months and the other group treated with inverse occlusion and given at least one hour of daily training, except on weekends, for an average of 8 weeks. Fixation was para- macular or peripheral in all but two cases in the former group and in all but one case in the latter group. Their results confirmed that oc- clusion of the sound eye proved superior to inverse occlusion in both fixation and acuity improvement in the age groups 3 to 6 and 6 to 9 and was equally successful in the age group 9 to 12. They also found no evidence that conventional occlusion intensified an existing eccen- tric fixation and they preferred this technique even in the oldest age group, since it was simpler to perform.

In analyzing these findings, it should be reiterated that the success of inverse occlusion depends primarily on the time devoted daily to fixation and acuity training and on the skill and effectiveness of its administration. Perhaps with the good patient cooperation and with more intensive daily training the reported results obtained with in- verse occlusion would have been better.

Another consideration is the type of fixation anomaly to be treated. It should be anticipated that the grosser and more variable fixation anomalies would respond more favorably to conventional occlusion than would the smaller, stable and fixed type.

It is apparent that conventional occlusion remains the method of choice for patients up to age 5 because such patients generally respond readily to routine occlusion. Children in this age group are usually too young to profit from the training which must accompany inverse occlusion, the use of which would result in the deterioration of fixation and acuity through the promotion of disuse.

Since conventional occlusion has been found not to intensify ec- centric fixation and since it is the simpler method to perform, it also remains the preferred initial approach, regardless of the type of fixa- tion, for patients older than age 4.

Inverse occlusion may be of value for those who do not respond to conventional occlusion, as a preliminary to conventional occlusion, for those intermittent periods during the day when conventional oc- clusion cannot be practiced due to locomotion hazards or inability to work, for small angle and stable eccentric fixation, or for older age groups when effective and intensive daily training can be provided.

Standard Occlusion

The occlusion practiced with the inverse technique is always total and constant; usable form and light are excluded during the waking hours. Standard occlusion, however, may be practiced in a number of ways, depending upon the nature of the problem. The methods vary in accordance with the time the occluder is worn, the manner in which it affects the transmission of light and form, and the way it is applied to the eye.

Occlusion may be classified according to time worn, such as constant (worn in front of one eye all day) and as periodic or part time (worn in front of one eye during prescribed periods of the day). It may be classified according to transmission characteristics, as follows:

(1) *Opaque:* the complete exclusion of a retinal image for the affected portion of the visual field through the use of an opaque material; termed *total occlusion* when completely eliminating both usable form and light, producing a monocular condition, or *partial occlusion* when excluding only selected portions of the visual field from stimulating the eye or eyes.

(2) *Translucent* (diffusing): the exclusion of usable form vision, but stimulation of the eye with diffused light, for the affected portion of the visual field, as accomplished with translucent plastic or by frosting or etching all or part of a glass spectacle lens.

(3) *Distorting:* the creation of a distorted retinal image of selected amount by means of an irregularly refracting lens to reduce visual acuity to a desired level.

(4) *Blurring:* the creation of an out-of-focus retinal image by means of a cycloplegic (usually atropine) or a spectacle lens of appropriate dioptric power to reduce visual acuity to a desired level.

(5) *Dimming* (obscuring): the creation of a dim retinal image with reduced contrast by restricting the amount of light entering the eye to reduce visual acuity to a desired level, as accomplished with a neutral filter of selected density, with paired Polaroid filters rotated to a selected axial relationship, or with plastic material of selected transparency.

(6) *Chromatic:* the creation of a retinal image of selected color content by means of a color filter (usually dark red).

OPAQUE AND TRANSLUCENT OCCLUSION
METHODOLOGY

Occlusion should be started as soon as possible, regardless of whether it is a preventive or a corrective measure. To be most effective, conventional occlusion should be practiced constantly in either opaque or translucent form; its purpose is to exercise the fixation reflex and to promote the cortical reception and interpretation of impulses from the amblyopic eye. The more hours of occlusion each day, the greater the stimulation and the faster and greater the improvement.

Either opaque or translucent occlusion completely neutralizes the occluded eye and affords maximum stimulation of the amblyopic eye by shifting the entire burden of visual identification to it.

Constant and total occlusion is more commonly employed than constant and translucent occlusion because the former, in eliminating all stimuli, is more easily tolerated. The diffused light which bathes the occluded eye in translucent occlusion may conflict with and rival, at least initially, the interpretation of the images from the nonoccluded eye. On occasion, it results in visual annoyance, headache and nausea. Results from translucent occlusion, however, compare favorably with those from opaque occlusion.

Two approaches to translucent occlusion offer a distinct cosmetic advantage over opaque occlusion in that the occluded eye remains visible even though form vision is completely obliterated. One method is to mask the back surface of the spectacle lens with Scotch brand Magic Tape; the other is to apply a thin coat of transparent nail polish rapidly and evenly to the back surface of a spectacle lens and pat it with the brush until dry, thereby imparting a stippled and frosted finish to the surface. In either case, the lens has a filmy or smudged appearance. The nail polish is easily removed with acetone.

A translucent plastic clip-on or an etched glass spectacle lens does not offer the same advantage, but either one is cosmetically superior to opaque occlusion.

Occlusion and Binocular Vision. Constant opaque or translucent occlusion provides the greatest and fastest improvement, but it should be prescribed only when one is certain that it will not produce undesirable side effects. Strabismic amblyopia in association with constant strabismus is the condition best suited for constant occlusion, but only if no peripheral fusion is evidenced and if occlusion is begun at a preschool age. Under these circumstances, constant occlusion will not disrupt or break down any fusion response, since none exists; the risk of breaking down a peripheral suppression response with subsequent and persistent diplopia after removal of the occluder is minimal. Problems involved in attending school and working are absent; patient cooperation is attained more readily; and patient exposure to jibes and taunts is reduced.

Should constant occlusion be attempted for the same condition later in life, the possibility of a constant diplopia increases; difficulties may be encountered in attending school or working may make it impractical: patient cooperation is attained less easily because adolescents and adults are less prone to comply with the dictates of parents or doctors; and the psychological trauma of wearing an occluder becomes more pronounced.

In addition to those accentuated problems, a further risk is present in the adult who has a condition characterized by cosmetically straight eyes, a case history of unilateral estropia with an apparent spontaneous reduction in the deviation, the continued persistence of amblyopia ex anopsia and suppression, and the complete absence of fusion. Prescribing constant occlusion in such an instance may not only result in constant diplopia but also may create a marked increase in the strabismic deviation, both of which are likely to persist.

If constant total or translucent occlusion is indicated in a child of school age—and if a problem exists because of a risk in walking to and from school or because of an inability to perform schoolwork or because school authorities will not permit the child on school grounds in this potentially hazardous condition—during this interim the occlusion may be shifted to the amblyopic eye. The purpose is to remove permanently the influence of suppression by always maintaining a monocular condition in order to facilitate the ultimate restoration of fusion. Ideally, it is best to start occlusion during the summer months, when such problems usually are absent and when the child is not exposed to the harassment of his schoolmates.

Constant translucent or opaque occlusion is contraindicated when binocular vision is present in some form as in anisometropic amblyopia unaccompanied by strabismus, in strabismic amblyopia associated with intermittent or periodic strabismus, or in strabismic amblyopia associated with a constant small-angle residual strabismus in which peripheral fusion is present, acting to overcome some but not all of the deviation. Creation of a monocular situation by constant occlusion, especially if it is prolonged, might succeed in breaking down the binocular response, producing constant strabismus.

If binocular vision is present in some form, translucent or opaque occlusion should be part time, or occlusion should be full time in the form of a blurring, distorting or dimming lens which reduces acuity in the occluded eye to a level significantly below that of the amblyopic eye. In the latter approach, binocular vision is permitted and at the same time increased use of the impulses from the amblyopic eye is encouraged.

Alternation of Occlusion. In conventional occlusion, the sound eye is occluded until it is established that maximum improvement has been attained. At this stage, in constant strabismus, constant total or translucent occlusion may be continued by alternating occlusion between the two eyes or by providing half occlusion of each spectacle lens (the nasal halves in esotropia and the temporal halves in exotropia).

The purpose of alternation is to maintain the fixation reflex and visual acuity at peak performance in both eyes and also to prevent the need for and use of suppression and anomalous correspondence. In so doing, the ultimate objective of establishing binocular fixation and normal sensory fusion is simplified. Alternation is typically performed on a daily schedule, one day one eye being occluded and the next day the other eye being occluded. This is in keeping with the stated purposes of occlusion: not only to foster improved fixation and visual acuity in an amblyopic eye but also to prevent the continued use of the anomalous binocular habits which exist in constant strabismus.

In the preventive care of preschool unilateral strabismics of recent onset, occlusion is alternated for the same purposes, but it is interspersed with brief periods of remission, such as occlusion three days a week followed by an equal period of no occlusion. The periods of remission are used to determine if binocular fixation and fusion can be attained spontaneously or through visual training (age and cooperation permitting) or through the help of a spectacle correction which may contain prism power to remove excessive demand on motor fusion. Remission from occlusion is of relatively short duration in order to prevent the formation or strengthening of adaptive anomalies.

Partial or Half Occluders.   Half occluders are sometimes used instead of alternating total occlusion to accomplish the same objectives, especially in large-angle strabismic deviations. Binasal occlusion is used more frequently in esotropia than is bitemporal occlusion in exotropia because, in the latter, the blocking of the temporal fields of vision poses a hazard. The principles of binasal or bitemporal occlusion are (1) to promote the alternation of fixation as objects in the right or left field of vision are fixated, since they are visible only to one or the other eye, (2) through alternation of fixation, to maintain acuity in the two eyes or to improve acuity in an amblyopic eye, (3) to eliminate the use of suppression and anomalous correspondence by blocking the field of the nonfixating eye as it deviates behind the occluder, (4) by using (2) and (3) to effect a reduction in strabismic deviation and (5) to permit the possibility of binocular fixation should there be a straightening of the eyes in constant strabismus or should this skill already be present.

These objectives can be achieved only if occlusion is properly applied to the spectacle lenses and if the patient fixates objects to the right or left by eye movements and not head movement. If head movement takes place despite instructions to the contrary, alternation of occlusion should be given to be certain that fixation is actively performed by each eye.

Half occluders are either opaque or translucent and may be made by applying masking tape to the ocular side of the spectacle lens, by applying stippled transparent nail polish or Scotch brand Magic Tape to the ocular surface of the spectacle lens, by using half occluder clip-ons, or by etching a glass spectacle lens. In designing the half occluders, measurements are made of the distance between the nasal margins of the pupils as each eye in turn fixates straight ahead for a distant target and for a near target. These two measurements determine the portions of each spectacle lens which remain free from occlusion (see Figure 14). Binocular fixation is possible, but only for the straight-ahead position.

Swenson (1953, 1958) recommends the use of temporal occlusion before the deviating eye in esotropia as a means of breaking down eccentric fixation and improving acuity in amblyopia and also to

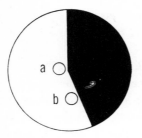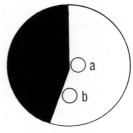

Figure 14. Binasal occlusion, as may be used in esotropia, the distance between the nasal margin of each pupil for straight ahead fixation of each eye at far (a) and near (b) determining the nasal limits of the occluder on each spectacle lens.

counteract suppression and anomalous correspondence. She applies opaque material to the temporal portion of the spectacle lens so that its nasal limit bisects the pupil of the deviating eye as the dominant eye fixates a light source in the midplane at a distance of 30 cm. Swenson claims that her method serves these purposes and even tends to decrease deviation, in some cases producing orthophoria.

OPAQUE AND TRANSLUCENT OCCLUDERS

Tape-Ons. The tape-on patch is used when total occlusion is desired and when spectacle lenses are not worn, or when a child will not cooperate with other forms of occlusion which are easily removed or which permits peeking around the sides.

The disadvantages of tape-ons include the tendency for the skin to become irritated by the continued and prolonged use of an adhesive and by the entrapment of body heat; the undesirability of keeping the eyelids constantly closed; the need to maintain an adequate supply of them because they usually must be discarded once removed; and their poor cosmetic appearance.

One of the best tape-ons is the Elastoplast Eye Occlusor (Duke Laboratories). This is a flesh-colored tape, oval in shape and containing a thin oval gauze pad at the center of its gummed surface, leaving only a narrow band exposed for taping to the orbital rim. The tape is designed to permit the passage of air and not to irritate the skin. It may be obtained in two sizes, Junior and Adult, in boxes of two dozen.

A ready-made gauze patch taped over the eye may also be used, but its thickness and the task of taping it to the face and removing it make it undesirable for prolonged use.

Tie-Ons. The tie-on is an opaque occluder available in ribbed cloth, in cupped plastic or rubber, and in black, frost, or flesh color. It is affixed to the head by an elastic band or by tying attached ribbons behind the head. This form of occluder is most frequently used when short periods of supervised occlusion are desired, as in testing or training. It may be used with an elastic band for constant occlusion for adults, but children dislodge or remove it too easily, and it is cosmetically objectionable.

Clip-Ons. The clip-on occluder is made in two forms: a patch clip-on, which covers only the spectacle lens and is clipped to its front surface, and a cup clip-on, which is clipped to the back surface of the spectacle lens and has peripheral extensions contouring, and in juxtaposition to, the nose, eyebrow, cheek and temple, to block peripheral vision.

The patch variety may be obtained in hard plastic in translucent form and in opaque black or flesh color. It is also available in opaque, flesh-colored soft plastic with metal clips, such as the Linder patch occluder (1) in Figure 15.

The hard plastic patch clip-on may be obtained in round or oval shape and in several sizes, usually from 36 mm to 46 mm, so as to relate properly to the spectacle lens. The Linder patch occluder comes in three sizes, 38 mm, 42 mm and 46 mm, and is preferred because its metal clips provide a more durable construction and it is less easily removed from the frame.

The translucent or the opaque hard plastic patch clip-on is frequently used for constant and prolonged occlusion, although it is better suited for brief occlusion intervals during testing or training.

The disadvantage of a patch clip-on, in addition to the ease with which it can be removed by an uncooperating child, is that the patient can use the occluded eye by peeking around the sides or by moving the spectacle frame down on the nose and looking over its top. If undetected, this could have a serious effect on the outcome because under such circumstances vision will not improve. This is especially so if the occlusion is not accompanied by active training.

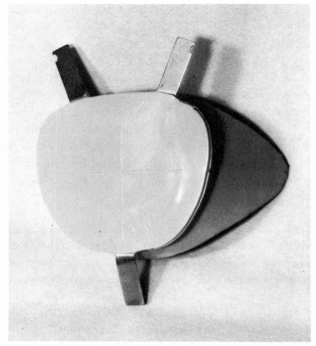

Figure 15. The Linder Cup occluder.

The cup clip-on, by completely blocking out all peripheral vision, is preferable to the patch clip-on. It may be obtained in hard plastic (Doyne Occluder: Bel-O-cluder), in soft flexible plastic with a cushioned rim (Pap Occluder), and in flesh-colored soft plastic with three flexible metal clips (Linder cup occluder) (1). The cup clip-on occluders are made for the right and left eyes and in several sizes.

The Linder cup occluder (Figure 15) is the most desirable because it may be easily trimmed to facial contours to ensure comfort, a point not to be overlooked when prescribing any cup clip-on. Flesh color is generally the most acceptable.

Suction Types. The suction occluder is similar to the cup clip-on, the only difference being that it is affixed to the posterior surface of the spectacle lens by means of a suction cup instead of clips. Examples of suction occluders are the Jamieson occluder, which is made of easily trimmed, flesh-colored soft rubber with a temporal opening for

ventilation, and the Vaccluder, which is made of plastic with an attached rubber suction cup, flesh colored on the outside and black on
the inside. They are cosmetically less desirable than clip-on cup
occluders and they are easily dislodged.

Masking. In this form of occlusion, a substance such as stippled
transparent nail polish, plastic foil, Scotch brand Magic Tape, masking
tape or adhesive tape is applied to selected portions or all of the surface of the spectacle lens to render it either translucent or opaque.
Stippled translucent nail polish and Scotch tape offer the cosmetic
advantage of permitting the occluded eye to be seen through the lens.
An etched glass lens may be used for translucent occlusion, but it requires a specially made lens and the eye cannot be seen through it.

Occasionally, an opposite approach to occlusion is taken: instead
of attempting to make the occluder as inconspicuous as possible, it is
made noticeable in some way, such as by painting a picture of an eye
on an opaque occluder. Adolescents are likely to improvise on their
occluders in this manner to make the best of an unpleasant situation.

Recognizing this aspect of occlusion, Bausch and Lomb (4) has
designed a variety of Cartoon Eye Patches available in sheets of
twelve for gumming to the anterior surface of the spectacle lens or to
an occluder (Figure 16). The patient may select the one (of a total
of twenty-eight) he finds most appealing.

If an emotional rebellion is encountered in accepting occlusion, one
may utilize a series of plastic foils of graded transparency (Bangerter's graded occluders) (17) to reduce vision gradually in the nonamblyopic eye until total occlusion is achieved. This method of initiating occlusion, named *sneak occlusion* by Bangerter, allows the child
to adapt slowly to reduced vision in the amblyopic eye. The plastic
foils are affixed to the spectacle lens and come in eight gradations of
density, designed to reduce vision in eight steps from approximately
20/30 to 20/200. The reverse procedure may be used when discontinuing occlusion, and the same calibrated occluders may be employed to
maintain a given reduction in the vision of the nonamblyopic eye in
order to encourage the use of the amblyopic eye while still permitting
binocular vision (as in treating anisometropic amblyopia).

Another approach used to gain a patient's acceptance of an occluder and the poor vision of the amblyopic eye is first to apply an
opaque occluder to the amblyopic eye to permit adaptation to the

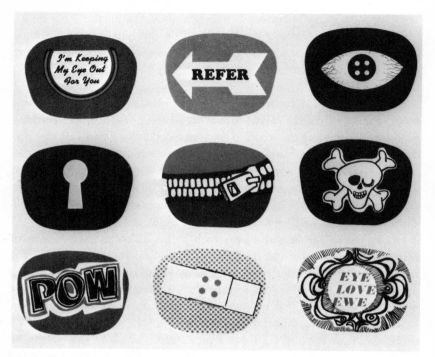

Figure 16. The Bausch and Lomb Cartoon Eye Patches.

wearing of the occluder. The occluder is then shifted to the non-amblyopic eye for gradually increasing periods each day until it it worn during all waking hours. When the nonamblyopic eye first receives occlusion for brief intervals, the child's activities should be confined to playing games with gross objects near so that reduced vision will not present a severe handicap and the initiation will occur under pleasant circumstances. Once that is achieved, the child may be permitted to walk about the house and eventually play outdoors.

Contact Lenses. From the cosmetic standpoint, the ideal way of achieving constant total occlusion is through the use of a contact lens rendered opaque centrally so as to block light completely from passing through the pupil. The time and expense required to fit such a lens, and the young age levels at which constant total occlusion is usually practiced, however, tend to make this method clinically impractical except under unusual circumstances.

DISTORTING OCCLUSION

By prescribing an irregularly refracting spectacle lens designed to produce a specified degree of distortion to the retinal image in the nonamblyopic eye, the patient's use of an amblyopic eye is encouraged while still permitting binocular vision. The amount of distortion should be sufficient to reduce visual acuity to at least two Snellen lines below that of the amblyopic eye in order to promote the use of the amblyopic eye for visual identification.

Cosmetically, the distorting lens is excellent; it appears to be an ordinary lens and the eye is seen normally through it. Functionally, it is superior to the presentation of an out-of-focus retinal image (as by overcorrecting in convex lenses) since the same degree of distortion is present at all fixation distances.

The Chavasse Lens (Scientype occluder) is an example of the distorting lens. It is available in two forms, one designed to reduce acuity to 20/200 and the other to reduce acuity to 20/1200. The Occluder Lens (1), also based on this principle, offers a selection in visual acuity reduction ranging from 20/100 to 20/1600. Occluder Lenses may be obtained in trial sets, enabling the clinical determination of the lens which will achieve a desired level of acuity reduction. They may also be obtained as partial occluders (Semi-Occluders), should half occluders be desired. A single occluder lens, pressed from a ball-peened mold and reducing visual acuity to 20/1200, is offered by Bausch and Lomb (4), but reducing acuity to such a low level, in effect, creates a monocular condition. A contact lens made of a plastic of uneven refractive index and designed to reduce acuity to 20/400 may also be used for this purpose (19).

BLURRING OCCLUSION

Another method of fostering the use of an amblyopic eye while still permitting binocular vision is to blur the retinal image of the non-amblyopic eye. The out-of-focus retinal image is obtained by prescribing a spectacle lens which over- or undercorrects in cylindrical power, which overcorrects in convex spherical power, or which undercorrects in concave spherical power. The amount of blur introduced is in accordance with the acuity reduction required, a minimum reduction being an acuity at least two Snellen lines below that of the amblyopic eye.

Departure in spherical power from the emmetropic prescription, however, does not ensure that the amblyopic eye will be favored for all distances of fixation. At near ranges, the nonamblyopic eye may offer superior acuity unless the amount of induced myopia is considerable, blurring vision below that of the amblyopic eye at routine, near working distances.

Blurred vision may also be accomplished through cycloplegia. Atropine or other cycloplegics, in manifesting latent hypermetropia and preventing accommodation, will result in a blur at both far and near distances. A disadvantage is that the amount of blur cannot be controlled, and as a result the nonamblyopic eye may continue to provide better vision than the amblyopic eye at both far and near distances, especially at far. Further, the continued and prolonged paralysis of the ciliary muscle is undesirable, and the dilation of the pupil may result in sensitivity to light.

Atropine may be used as a means of initiating total occlusion by promoting the use of the amblyopic eye prior to occlusion of the nonamblyopic eye. Johnson and Antuna (1965) have reported good acuity improvement in amblyopia associated with accommodative esotropia by using atropine on the dominant eye and a miotic (Phospholine Iodide) on the amblyopic eye. The combined use of a cycloplegic on the fixating eye and a miotic on the amblyopic eye appeared to be more effective in restoring normal vision to the amblyopic eye than the use of a cycloplegic alone.

DIMMING (OBSCURING) OCCLUSION

The favoring of the amblyopic eye over the normally fixating eye in the presence of binocular stimulation may be attained by reducing the amount of light entering the fixating eye. By controlling the amount of light entering the nonamblyopic eye (graded or calibrated occlusion), the visual acuity may be reduced to a desired level, promoting the use of the amblyopic eye for all distances of fixation.

The simplest method of regulating light transmission is through the use of neutral filters attached to the spectacle lens. The Pugh occluders (Pugh's Visual Acuity Reducers) serve this purpose and consist of a series of four clip-on neutral filters of different densities.

These filters, however, still permit fairly good acuity, the most dense providing an acuity of approximately 20/60. Ruben's Selective Occluder (6) also utilizes neutral filters which are held in place in front of the eye by means of a sleeve fitted over the temple and front of the spectacle frame. The neutral filter comes in sheet form, is cut in strips for individual use, and is used in multiple layers, the number of layers dictated by the acuity reduction desired.

Kodak Wratten neutral density filters, Bangerter's graded occluders. and gray-tinted contact lenses may be similarly employed. Light transmission may also be reduced by using paired clip-on Polaroid filters, rotated to a desired axes relationship. That technique, however, is of value primarily for testing or training rather than for constant wear.

CHROMATIC OCCLUSION

Color filters serve many useful purposes in the testing and training of visual functions; in amblyopia ex anopsia, occlusion with a dark red filter may be useful in breaking down eccentric fixation, in improving visual acuity, and in removing suppression influences.

In the Humphriss method (1937), a red filter is placed in front of the nonamblyopic eye for gradually increasing periods each day and the patient is encouraged to attempt to see objects as normally colored instead of red. As long as the nonamblyopic eye dominates in fixation and cortical attention, objects will continue to be seen as red, but when the amblyopic eye assumes fixation, objects will appear normally colored. The patient's insight in realizing that objects will continue to appear red as long as the amblyopic eye is ignored, combined with the unpleasantness of seeing everything as red, particularly while eating, serves as the motivating force in promoting the use of the amblyopic eye. Another aspect, not considered at the time by Humphriss, is that the red filter also has a dimming effect, lessening the effectiveness of the retinal image of the nonamblyopic eye by reducing the amount of light transmitted and causing the eye to become dark adapted. If the technique is successful, the patient will experience interspersed moments of normal colors which gradually increase in duration until they predominate.

Brinker and Katz (1963) have advocated a method for treating eccentric fixation in which the nonamblyopic eye is totally occluded and a red filter which excludes wavelengths shorter than 640 millimicrons

(Kodak gelatin Wratten filter No. 92) is placed in front of the amblyopic eye. The procedure is carried out until fixation becomes centric and is then followed by conventional occlusion without the red lens.

The method is based on the assumption that, although the eye becomes dark adapted, the cone cells concentrated in the fovea remain sensitive to the extreme red end of the spectrum while the rod cells are insensitive to this spectral region. With the rod cells insensitive to wavelengths longer than 640 millimicrons, the use of the fovea with its cone cells would be encouraged, and fixation with a more peripheral portion of the retina containing primary rod cells would be discouraged. This stimulative condition would then afford a means of combating gross eccentric fixation.

The theoretical basis proposed by Brinker and Katz, however, is incorrect. Although in dark adaptation the scotopic luminosity curve is shifted by approximately 50 millimicrons toward the short end of the spectrum, compared to the photopic luminosity curve (Purkinje's phenomenon), the threshold sensitivities of rods and cones for wavelengths longer than 640 millimicrons are essentially equal (Adler, 1963, 1965).

Despite that error, Brinker and Katz reported success in breaking down eccentric fixation and in improving visual acuity, the time required ranging from 6 to 14 weeks. Favorable results were also obtained by others (Binder et al., 1963; Kunst, 1963; Ratiu and Reiter, 1966; Cowle, Kunst and Philpotts, 1967), but improvement tended to be slow and incomplete with best results in children younger than 5, the age group which generally responds well to simple conventional occlusion.

The reported improvements may be related to the amount of light transmitted and to the resulting dark-adapted state of the amblyopic eye, rather than to wavelength transmitted. In amblyopia ex anopsia, the amblyopic eye improves in both visual acuity and fixation responses when dark adapted.

Other red filters found satisfactory for this procedure include the Kodak gelatin Wratten filter No. 25, which transmits wavelengths between 580 and 700 millimicrons, with a luminous transmittance of 22.5 percent (Cowle et al., 1967), and the Ruby Kodaloid filter (Binder et al., 1963), which has almost the same transmission characteristics as the Kodak Wratten filter No. 92 but is more durable.

In using the Brinker-Katz method, to stimulate the amblyopic eye solely with red light, an opaque side shield should be used to block out peripheral white light. Indoors, care should be taken to provide sufficient light to enable adequate awareness of objects. Because of the poor cosmetic appearance and the distaste of seeing everything in red, increased patient resistance may be anticipated, especially when acuity is poor. These disadvantages tend to limit the use of this training approach to a few hours a day, as when conducting other training.

Doctor-Patient Relationships

INDOCTRINATION

Two factors may cause a patient to rebel against wearing an occluder: the cosmetic handicap and the poor acuity afforded by the amblyopic eye. The more unsightly the occluder and the poorer the acuity in the amblyopic eye, the more intense is the problem. These two serious hurdles should be fully recognized. When prescribing occlusion, all possible steps should be taken to gain the acceptance and cooperation of both the patient and his parents.

When recommending occlusion for a child, the child should not be present. Not infrequently, the parents' first reaction is one of dismay; if the child is present and observes his parents' unhappiness, he will take it to mean that occlusion is something "bad" and that his parents do not want him to have it. Encouraged by their display of displeasure and reluctance, his cooperation will be just that much more difficult to obtain.

The parents (or the adult patient) should be told why occlusion is necessary and how important it is to follow this recommendation. They should also be cautioned against displaying resentment in the child's presence and should be advised to warn their relatives and neighbors to take the same precaution.

Once parent insight and willingness are attained, the child should be told what is being planned and why. It can be demonstrated, even to a 3-year-old, that one eye does not see as well as the other. This demonstration may be followed by such statements as: "Now I know you don't want to go around letting one eye do all the work!" or "Now

I know you would like to have this eye see as well as the other eye!" or "We can make this lazy eye get to work and see as well as the other eye, and I know you would like that!"

The Bangerter innovation of confining amblyopic patients to a "school" while practicing occlusion and providing training is the ideal solution to the problem of patient acceptance. Not only can properly supervised training be given several hours each day, but the wearing of an occluder is also met with a minimum of resistance since all the "schoolmates" are wearing one. If it were readily available and accepted by an educated public, the training school concept would greatly simplify the treatment of amblyopia as well as other visual training problems.

We have seen that the best techniques used to introduce a patient to occlusion include the initial patching of the amblyopic eye, prior to conventional occlusion, to familiarize the patient with occlusion, later shifting the occluder to the nonamblyopic eye for gradually increasing periods; confining the initial wearing of the occluder to short periods of time during which simple training games are performed at close range, gradually increasing the wearing time with restriction limited to indoor wear, and eventually increasing to full-time wear; using the "sneak occlusion" method in which a series of filters of successively increasing density are used until total occlusion is achieved; and performing occlusion during vacation when the child is not attending school so as not to interfere with schoolwork and to minimize exposure to other children. Translucent occluders are cosmetically superior to opaque occluders, and in the latter a flesh color is more acceptable than black. A contact lens occluder presents no cosmetic problem, nor do dimming, distorting or blurring occluders.

Intense and persistent opposition may be encountered to the wearing of an opaque or translucent occluder if the visual acuity in the amblyopic eye is 20/200 or lower. With such poor acuity, the child is severely handicapped, and immediate and continued rebellion is understandable, especially in young children. An extreme, adverse reaction that persists requires the discontinuance of occlusion until the child is older and more likely to cooperate.

It should also be realized that, in amblyopia ex anopsia, acuity reductions are seldom less than 20/200 and that acuities lower than 20/200 very likely are of congenital or pathological origin, in which case occlusion and training cannot help.

INTERIM OBSERVATION

During occlusion, fixation and acuity of the amblyopic eye and of the occluded eye should be checked weekly. This is especially necessary in young children when no office training is being conducted. Occlusion amblyopia may occur quickly between ages 1 and 3 and one must be on the alert for its development. If detected, occlusion should be reversed for a brief interval and then alternated to ensure the maintenance of normal vision in both eyes.

If no improvement is made after a reasonable period of occlusion, it should be ascertained if the child is cooperating in wearing the occluder and is performing the training. Frequently, close questioning will reveal whether or not the child is peeking around the occluder, or taking it off, and not making an effort to accomplish his training tasks. The parents may be more to blame for this than the child; although the importance of following instructions is stressed, they frequently are negligent in supervising the wearing of the occluder and fail to devote the time or to exhibit the patience required in home training.

Pleasure should be demonstrated and the child praised for his good work if acuity increases, in order to encourage both the patient and his parents to continue their efforts. Prizes may also be given to the child.

Care should be taken in reevaluating acuity to test in the same manner as that performed originally, measuring both line and single-letter acuity without extra urging or prompting and by using the same percentage of correct responses as was the criterion for designating acuity.

DURATION OF TRAINING

The rate and extent of improvement through occlusion will vary with the age of onset, the age at which treatment begins, the constancy with which occlusion is practiced, patient and parent cooperation, the existence or absence of eccentric fixation, and whether or not effective training is performed concurrently.

Rapid improvement will occur if constant opaque or translucent occlusion is carried out at preschool ages, when the visual mechanism is pliable and the child likely to cooperate. Normal fixation and normal acuity will return in a few weeks, or even sooner, age 1 responding is pliable and the child likely to cooperate. Normal fixation and norfaster than age 2 and age 2 responding faster than age 3 or 4. Improvement will be comparatively slow if occlusion begins after this age level, the same trend still continuing, however, ages 5 to 8 responding better than ages 9 to 12, and adults showing both the slowest rate and smallest degree of improvement, the attainment of 20/20 being rare.

At these relatively older ages, eccentric fixation becomes a greater problem and cooperation is attained less easily. Further, in addition to occlusion, an intensive training program must be followed to achieve maximum improvement. Depending on these factors, it may take from several weeks to several months before no further improvement is noted, the likelihood of achieving 20/20 vision diminishing with advancing age and acuities between 20/25 and 20/40 being more typical.

In patients aged 5 to 12, occlusion performed constantly and faithfully, especially if accompanied by visual training, generally results in an acuity improvement within 2 weeks, with maximum improvement reached in from 4 to 8 weeks. Near vision may improve faster than distance vision, and this may serve as a clue to subsequent improvement of distance vision (Enos, 1944; Kramer, 1953).

Should part-time occlusion be practiced for any of the reasons previously cited, progress will be slower. It is imperative when performing part-time occlusion that concentrated training be provided during the periods the occluder is worn in order to provide sufficient stimulation to realize an improvement. Further, the occluder should be worn for as many hours each day as is feasible; an hour or two each day is insufficient.

Unilateral occlusion should be continued until normal fixation and acuity are present or until no further improvement is manifested. In the latter instance, to be certain that no further improvement is possible, occlusion should be practiced for an additional few weeks. If after this time the condition remains stable, occlusion can be discontinued either abruptly or gradually.

In constant strabismus, occlusion can now be alternated between the two eyes or half occluders can be used to prevent the use of binocular anomalies and to maintain acuity and fixation in both eyes. This type of occlusion is continued until normal binocular vision is established or until training to eliminate the strabismus proves unsuccessful.

For acuity and fixation improvements to become permanent, normal binocular vision either must be present or, if constant strabismus persists, it must be alternating, with the formerly amblyopic eye participating in the act of fixation.

If no change in vision is apparent after several weeks of faithfully practiced constant occlusion, it is likely that the anomaly is not one of amblyopia ex anopsia and occlusion should be discontinued.

CHAPTER 18

Active Training Programs

Whether inverse or conventional occlusion is practiced, an active training program should be initiated concurrently in patients age 4 or older. The technique of inverse occlusion, of course, depends upon an intensive training program to stimulate actively the amblyopic eye, while the stimulation afforded by conventional occlusion is insufficient and should be supplemented by exacting training tasks specifically designed to foster improvement in a given skill or function.

The time saved by providing training along with conventional occlusion may be considerable. François and James (1955), in treating two groups of strabismic amblyopes of approximately the same ages, found that the group which received constant total occlusion and training attained the same level of improvement in less than one third of the time required by the group which received only constant total occlusion. This significant acceleration in attaining maximal results was accomplished by only two 1-hour training periods a week for 4 weeks. A more concentrated program would be expected to provide even more rapid results.

A variety of effective training techniques and procedures are available to treat the anomalies and deficiencies present in amblyopia ex anopsia, some complex and more suitably administered in the office or hospital, as those for eccentric fixation, and some simple and applicable to home training.

Bangerter's Method

To cope with the problem of amblyopia ex anopsia, Alfred Bangerter (1953, 1955) devised a concentrated and rigorous training program which he named *pleoptics* (derived from the Greek *pleon*, meaning full or complete, and *optikos*, meaning of or pertaining to sight), a term now popularly used as more or less synonymous with amblyopia training. The technique is based on the assumption that, due to inhibition of the central impulses, foveal sensitivity is reduced below that of the surrounding retina and that this in turn leads to eccentric fixation.

The procedure attempts to render the foveal area more sensitive than the surrounding retina (1) by depressing the sensitivity of either the site of eccentric fixation or an annular area around the fovea by "dazzling" and scotomizing it with a steady bright white light while shielding the fovea, (2) by stimulating the foveal area with a bright flashing light to build up synaptic relays and cortical reception, (3) by briefly repeating step 1, and (4) by providing a series of monocular fixation drills which are performed immediately after the peripheral light stimulation in step 3 when the fovea is presumably more receptive to fixation stimuli. The fixation exercises are associated with, and take advantage of, other sense modalities, incorporating auditory, tactile, and memory clues to augment visual perception.

If eccentric fixation is present and persists after a brief trial period of conventional occlusion, inverse occlusion is given, commencing at least one month prior to the training and continuing between training periods until centric fixation is demonstrated. Conventional occlusion is then given and continued until maximum results are attained or until binocular skills have been established.

As conceived by Bangerter, the training is performed at a Pleoptic-Orthoptic school where the patients live or to which they go daily. Two 1-hour sessions are given each day for a period of 3 to 4 weeks. If indicated, the "term" may be repeated two to four times after an interval of rest.

Age 5 is considered the youngest at which cooperation may be attained, but, of course, the younger the age at which the training may be effectively performed, the better the prognosis. If eccentric fixation persists after four "terms," the training is discontinued.

LIGHT STIMULATION INSTRUMENTS

Originally, Bangerter attempted to provide the preliminary and preparatory light stimulation by means of a diaphragm-controlled lamp followed by stimulation with either a modified Gullstrand ophthalmoscope, adapted with a flashing device and a synchronized auditory stimulus, or a modified slit lamp adapted with a metronome to interrupt the light stimulation rhythmically. This instrumentation was eventually discarded in favor of a modified Nordenson fundus camera, which provided both a more intense light source and a view of the fundus which enabled precise localization of the light stimuli. Finally, Bangerter designed a new instrument, the Pleoptophor (Figure 17), to serve this purpose.

The Pleoptophor. The Pleoptophor is a table-mounted instrument which includes features of an indirect ophthalmoscope and fundus camera. It has two primary components: a system which illuminates and projects targets onto the fundus of the amblyopic eye, and a telescopic system, providing 18x magnification and a 40-degree field of view, through which the fundus is continuously observed during treatment. On either side of the telescope is a collimating system through which the right or left untreated eye views an adjustable fixation target. The fixation target is guided by the operator so that the fovea of the amblyopic eye becomes centered in, and encircled by, the projected targets. Illumination is variable, and a head clamp se-

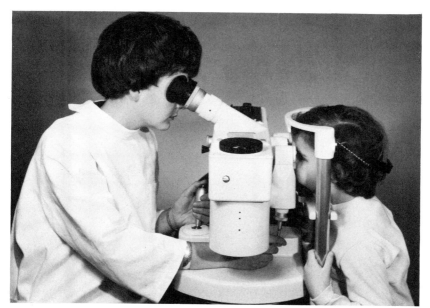

Figure 17. The Pleoptophor. (*Reprinted by permission of FISBA Optical Precision-Instruments Ltd., St. Gallen, Switzerland.*)

cures the patient's head in a fixed position. A mydriatic is advised to enable easy and constant view of the fundus.

The light stimulation with the Pleoptophor begins with the *dazzling phase,* in which the fovea is centered in the projected shadow of an opaque circular target, to shield it from illumination, while the remainder of the retina is stimulated for approximately 1 minute by intense light. The size of the opaque spot target depends on the magnitude of the eccentric fixation, 0.5 mm for parafoveal fixation, 1.0 mm for paramacular fixation, and 2.0 mm for peripheral fixation, corresponding to an angular subtense of 1 degree 40 minutes, 3 degrees 21 minutes, and 6 degrees 42 minutes, respectively (Figure 18). Once the fovea is centered in the shadow, a button is depressed which increases the illumination of the retina to a high intensity; its release, after the appropriate time interval, restores the original intensity. An alternative method may be used if eccentric fixation is steady. Dazzling is restricted to the eccentric site by presenting to the amblyopic eye (the other eye being occluded) a 2.0 mm, ring-shaped target with a 1.0 mm

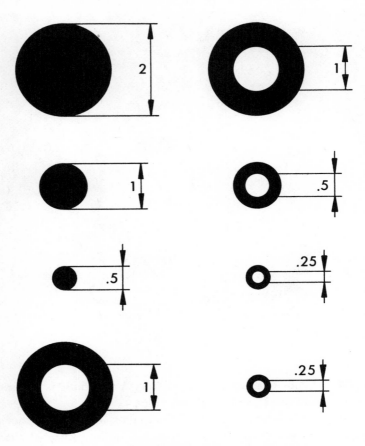

Figure 18. Stencils of targets used with the Pleoptophor in the dazzling phase (left) and the stimulative phase (right). The lower left and right targets are used when eccentric fixation is steady. Scaling is in millimeters.

open center (Figure 18). The amblyopic eye fixates the clear central area, and thus the eccentric site is exposed to the intense light.

The purpose of the dazzling phase is to depress the sensitivity of the eccentric site or of the peripheral retina and thereby relatively increase the receptiveness of the central retina. No emphasis is placed upon the presence of an afterimage.

The dazzling phase is immediately followed by the *stimulative phase*, in which the central area is stimulated by a series of 50 to 100 brief flashes of light. The target used for this phase consists of a polarizing filter containing an opaque ring with a clear center. The fovea is positioned so that it is encircled by the shadow of the opaque ring and will thus be exposed to the flashing light while an annular area around it is now shielded from the light. The diameter of the opaque ring is the same as that of the spot target used in the dazzling phase. In the alternate method of treating steady eccentric fixation, the target used in the stimulative phase has a 0.5-mm diameter and a 0.25-mm open center. The purpose of this phase is to stimulate the central pathway and reinforce synaptic relays and cortical reception.

The procedure with the Pleoptophor may be repeated two to four times per training session, the effects of each exposure lasting several minutes.

The Projectoscope. In lieu of the Pleoptophor, a sequence of like stimulation may be provided by the Nutt Auto-disc attachment for the Keeler Projectoscope (Figure 19). The Auto-disc is a small device

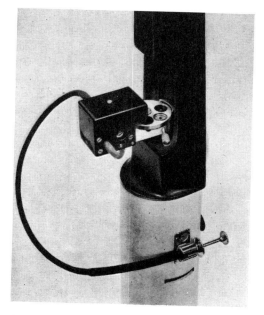

Figure 19. The Nutt Auto-disc mounted over the focusing tube of the Projectoscope. (*Reprinted by permission of Keeler Optical Products Ltd., Berkshire, England.*)

housing three graticules which are sequentially projected onto the fundus, the first being a green filter with a 3-degree lighter green center (or Linksz star), the second, a clear filter with a 3-degree central black dot, and the third, a dark green filter with a 1.5-degree clear central aperture (Bangerter's graticule).

. The attachment is fixed over the focusing tube of the instrument and cocked to preset the first graticule in position; with the untreated eye fixating a distant target, the light green center (or Linksz star) is positioned about the fovea of the amblyopic eye.

By pressing an attached cable release, the second graticule is rotated into position, the shadow of the black spot shielding the fovea; simultaneously, the control unit, to which the instrument is connected, boosts the illumination for a preset duration to provide an intense light stimulation to the unshielded retina (the dazzle phase). The plunger is depressed until the intense light stimulation is completed. Upon its release, the third graticule automatically rotates into position, the clear aperture now being centered about the fovea, and, simultaneously, the flash mechanism of the control unit is activated to provide a flashing light with a preset light and dark phase.

An individually mounted Bangerter graticule may also be used to provide just the stimulative phase, by placing it over the focusing tube (instead of the Auto-disc) and activating the flash mechanism.

The Projectoscope is not nearly as ideal as the Pleoptophor. Since it is hand held, it is difficult to maintain the proper positioning of the targets. Also, special arrangements are necessary to provide a fixation target for the untreated eye, so that the treated eye is easily accessible and the operator's head will not block the view of the untreated fixating eye.

TRAINING INSTRUMENTS

The preparatory stimulation with the Pleoptophor or Projectoscope (sometimes referred to as the passive phase), is immediately followed by the active phase, in which a variety of monocular training tasks are presented to the amblyopic eye to promote centric fixation and improve visual acuity.

Bangerter has devised a number of instruments for this purpose, but the training need not be confined to them; many other instruments may be used to accomplish the same objectives.

The Localizer. According to the Bangerter technique, the Localizer is one of the first instruments to be used, primarily to establish centric fixation and correct spatial localization. It consists of a flat face plate containing several small, countersunk, individually controlled lights, over which is placed one of a series of perforated plates. The openings, which are of a different diameter in each plate, are positioned directly above the light sources.

The patient fixates an illuminated opening with his amblyopic eye, and the position of the corneal reflex is noted to determine if fixation is centric (this by comparing the position of the corneal reflex to that which it occupies on the nonamblyopic eye when it fixates). If it is deemed eccentric, fixation is directed to a pointer held by the operator and the pointer is moved in the appropriate direction until the corneal reflex appears in the correct location.

The patient is now asked to touch the lighted opening with his finger while maintaining his eye in the directed position. The feel of the depression with the finger serves as a tactile clue to its location. Smaller illuminated openings are used for fixation targets as fixation improves, and the patient localizes the opening with a pointer instead of with his finger. The finger or pointer should be held slightly below, and close to, the fixating eye, aligned with the target, and then moved straight to it. The room illumination, which was originally dim, is raised to a normal level as increased skill is demonstrated.

It was pointed out in Chapter 12 that the dependence on the corneal reflex to detect eccentric fixation offers a poor means of interpretating a fixation response. The corneal reflex method is valid only if fixation is grossly eccentric and then only if the observer's eye is positioned directly above the fixated light source. In this training procedure, the observer is probably looking downward at the seated patient's eye, which in turn is looking downward at the illuminated hole. This would compound the difficulty of making a valid judgment as to the centricity of fixation. It would appear that greater reliance is placed on the light stimulation from the Pleoptophor to induce a centric fixation response than on the operator's observations and directions.

The Corrector. The Corrector is an instrument with which hand-eye coordination and spatial localization are stressed. It consists of a face plate over which is placed one of a series of metal plates containing insulated, grooved dots of various diameters or line drawings of gradually increasing complexity. The task of the patient is to fixate monocularly and contact, or trace over, the target with a hand-held metal stylus. Should the patient miss or stray off the target and the stylus contact the metal plate, an electric circuit is completed, causing a light to flash or a buzzer to sound. This alerts the patient to his error and to the necessity of making a corrective movement. As improvement is shown, the task is made harder. Consistent errors indicate the persistence of eccentric fixation, with its accompanying anomalous spatial localization, and the need to revert back to the Localizer to improve further fixation response.

The Localizer-Corrector. A commercially available instrument, the Localizer-Corrector, combines the features of the Localizer and Corrector (Figure 20). A single flat face plate is used interchangeably, either for one of five Localizer plates or for five Corrector plates. Each Localizer plate contains a picture with ten single-sized circular openings, ranging in diameter in the five plates from 5 mm to 1 mm. A clear plastic plate is also supplied which is placed over a Localizer plate to remove the tactile clue derived from the pointer when it contacts the rim of the opening.

In using the Corrector plates, a buzzer sounds and a light goes on if the metal stylus contacts the metal plate bordering the insulated target.

The Centrophor. The purpose of the Centrophor is to improve on an unsteady centric fixation or to reinforce a centric fixation. It is used immediately after treatment with the Pleoptophor. The Centrophor contains a target centered in a rotating spiral, both of which are viewed monocularly through a collimating system. The rotating spiral is intended to increase concentration and attention on the target at its center and thus promote a steady centric fixation. The size change induced by the motion afterimage created by the Plateau spiral effect does not enter into the training. A variety of independently illuminated targets may be used, as single or multiple letters, and the illumination of the spiral, which is at a maximum at the start, is gradually reduced until the target becomes distinct. A blue filter may also be used to create Haidinger's brushes, which are to be centered in the spiral. The speed of rotation of the spiral may be varied, the

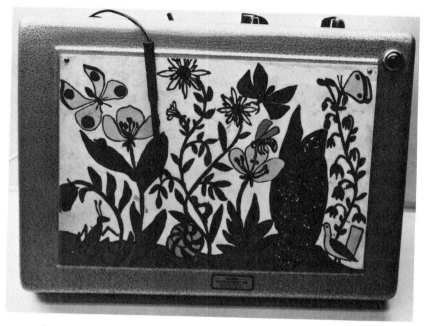

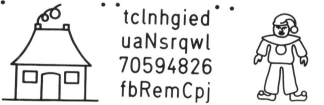

Figure 20. The Localizer-Corrector with Localizer plate (mounted on instrument) and Corrector plates.

speed and direction of rotation of Haidinger's brushes may be varied, and the visual angle of the image of the fixation target may be varied from 10 to 50 minutes of arc.

The Drill. The Drill is a table-mounted instrument containing a pointer mounted in a vertical tube which may be raised or lowered by an attached lever. It is designed to train hand-eye coordination and spatial localization. A plate containing several holes of various sizes is placed on a platform beneath the pointer. The patient monocularly aligns one hole with the pointer so that the pointer, when lowered, will pass through it without touching the sides, a buzzer sounding if the side is touched.

The Vibrating Localizer. Both the auditory and tactile senses are used with the Vibrating Localizer to assist visual perception in obtaining correct spatial localization. This small, hand-held instrument produces a vibration and a buzzing sound which furnishes clues as to its location when held, out of view, against one side of a screen (Figure 21). The patient, on the other side of the screen, attempts to

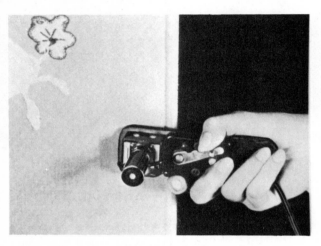

Figure 21. The Vibrating Localizer. (*Reprinted from Bangerter:* Amblyopiebehandlung, *1953, by permission of S. Karger, Basel/New York.*)

touch the region of the screen from which the sound is emanating, feeling a vibration if successful. After correct localization is demonstrated with the auditory clue, a light on the instrument is turned on to provide a visual clue. When correct localization is demonstrated with the added visual clue, the auditory and tactile clues are eliminated, leaving only the light as a means of determining its location.

The Acoustic Localizer. Spatial localization and hand-eye coordination are also trained with the Acoustic Localizer. An attempt is made to place a pointer into a monocularly fixated illuminated hole. A magnetic field acts to guide the pointer to the hole, as does the auditory clue of a humming sound which increases as the target is approached, ceasing when it is contacted.

The Mnemoscope. The Mnemoscope is a device which projects the image of a target onto a mirror, which in turn reflects it downward onto a stage where it is viewed by the amblyopic eye (Figure 22). The patient either traces over the image or duplicates it from memory. The illumination, exposure time, and projected image size may all be varied in accordance with the patient's acuity and skill.

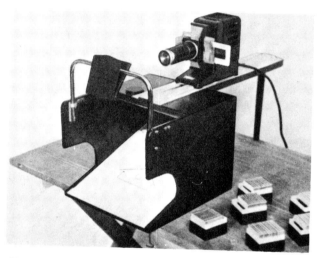

Figure 22. The Mnemoscope. (*Reprinted from Banger-ter:* Amblyopiebehandlung, *1953, by permission of S. Karger, Basel/New York.*)

The object of this training is to improve visual acuity through the assistance of visual memory. It is given when fixation is, or becomes, centric. The targets are presented in series, each series consisting of a group of slides, all containing the same picture but in decreasing size. Five such groups of targets are used, each succeeding group containing pictures of increasing complexity to represent five levels of difficulty.

The training begins by presenting the largest target of the simplest series, which is followed in sequence by gradually smaller versions of the same picture. The initial image size should be within the visual capability of the amblyopic eye. The patient reproduces the image of each exposure, the visual memory of the preceding larger image serving as a clue in identifying and reproducing the smaller version. After successful completion of the first series, the next more difficult series is exposed, the procedure being continued until all five groups have been accurately reproduced.

The Mnemoscope Trainer. The Mnemoscope Trainer also utilizes memory as a clue to visual perception and identification. The instrument consists of a long rectangular box, housing at one end a mirror system for reflecting the image of a target through an aperture where it is viewed by the amblyopic eye. The target is supported by a holder mounted on a track so that the viewing distance may be varied.

Visual acuity improvement is sought by presenting a target, such as a letter of the alphabet, at a viewing distance at which it is just identifiable, and then gradually increasing this distance. The patient strives to maintain recognition of the target as its image size is decreased.

The Letter Separator. Recognizing the accentuated crowding phenomenon, or separation difficulty, in strabismic amblyopia, Bangerter devised an instrument, the Letter Separator, or Surface Separation Trainer (Figure 23), to attack this problem and improve visual acuity. The key feature of this instrument is that the separation

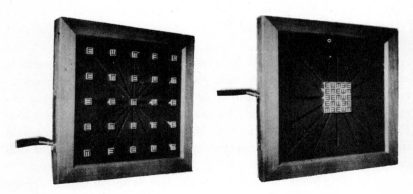

Figure 23. The Letter Separator. (*Reprinted by permission of the Omega Instrument Co., New York, N. Y.*)

of targets may be varied from approximately three target widths to juxtaposition. Twenty-five equal-sized and randomly orientated Snellen Es are mounted in radial slits on a vertical surface in square formation, the radial slits extending from a common center at 22.5-degree intervals. The separation of the Es is controlled by a lever at the side of the instrument.

The training starts with the Es maximally separated and at a fixation distance enabling correct identification of the direction of orientation. As the targets are gradually moved closer together, the patient is required to determine the orientation with each incremental decrease in target separation, which may be varied by the operator. This is continued until the Es are in juxtaposition, forming a solid square.

A newer version, the *Separator Trainer,* includes the factor of illumination of neighboring targets. This device consists of a box containing an internal light system and, on one of its vertical faces, 64 equal-sized Snellen Es, randomly orientated and in block formation. A plug-in arrangement, on another vertical face, enables the selective full illumination of any one of the Es, and a rheostat control enables the illumination of the neighboring targets to be varied from zero to that of the fixation target (Figure 24). The separation of the Es is not variable, but horizontal or vertical masking stripes may be used to block alternate rows from view, thereby varying the distance between targets and simplifying the task.

The patient views the Es at a distance at which the orientation may be just discerned when only the fixation target is illuminated. The illumination of the surrounding Es is then gradually increased. The ultimate accomplishment is the correct identification of the orientation of the plugged-in Es when the surrounding Es are maximally illuminated and contour interaction is in full effect. When this has been successfully performed, the procedure may be repeated at increased fixation distances.

HOME TRAINING

If the child does not reside at the "school" and if fixation is centric, a variety of simple monocular fixation and acuity exercises (such as tracing, coloring and sewing) is given as homework to accelerate improvement.

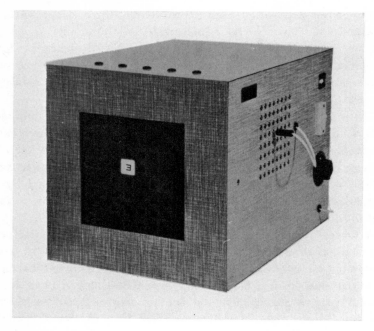

Figure 24. The Separator Trainer. (*Reprinted by permission of A. O. Ryser of Ryser Optiker, St. Gallen, Switzerland.*)

BINOCULAR TRAINING

When fixation is, or becomes, centric and visual acuity in the amblyopic eye is better than 20/50, orthoptic training is given at the "school" to eliminate strabismus. These techniques follow the conventional approaches and are beyond the scope of this text.

PREPLEOPTIC CARE

Realizing the importance of treating amblyopia ex anopsia at the earliest possible age, Bangerter intermittently atropinizes the fixating eye in infants who demonstrate constant unilateral strabismus in order to reduce the effectiveness of the fixating eye and encourage use of the deviating eye. Should this prove unsatisfactory, an alternative approach used in children below age 3 or 4 is to occlude the fixating eye, if fixation is not steady eccentric, employing the "sneak occlusion" technique. If amblyopia remains, pleoptic treatment starts as soon as the child is old enough to cooperate.

Prior to sneak occlusion or training, strabismus surgery is performed if the deviation is large (over 25 degrees), and the ametropia is corrected.

Cüppers' Method

The renewed interest created by Bangerter in the diagnosis and treatment of amblyopia ex anopsia prompted Curt Cüppers (1956) to devise new techniques to manage eccentric fixation and improve visual acuity. Unlike Bangerter, Cüppers does not believe that reduced sensitivity of the central retina leads to eccentric fixation. He attributes eccentric fixation in strabismic amblyopia to a perversion of the directional values in the amblyopic eye. This perversion is considered to be related to a preexisting anomalous correspondence which results, even under monocular conditions, in a shift of the principal (straight ahead) visual direction from the foveal center of the amblyopic eye to another retinal area. The retinal area which has acquired the principal visual direction is now used for monocular fixation in place of the foveal center.

Cüppers' training approach to attain centric fixation, therefore, lays emphasis on teaching the association of the straight ahead directional value with the foveal center. Eccentric fixation, and its resulting anomalous spatial localization, is made known to the patient by the projection and localization of negative afterimages or Haidinger's brushes, in relation to a monocularly fixated target. The negative afterimage, created by light stimulation of the retinal area peripheral to the fovea or macula, or the Haidinger's brushes, created by viewing a rotating Polaroid filter through a deep blue filter, will not be perceived to be centered about a fixation target if eccentric fixation is present. During training, the patient is taught to center the afterimage or brushes about the fixation target by making a corrective eye movement. If the training is successful, the amblyopic eye will eventually demonstrate an immediate centric fixation, as shown by the centering of the negative afterimage or brushes about the fixation point, without the necessity of corrective eye movements.

Cüppers agrees with Bangerter in advocating inverse occlusion for several weeks prior to training, if eccentric fixation is present, and the continuance of this occlusion, except for the training sessions, until fixation is centric. Occlusion of the nonamblyopic eye is practiced when fixation becomes centric or is centric at the outset.

Patients receiving training are confined to a hospital for a period of 3 to 6 weeks. The training is given twice daily, for one-hour periods. Since the tasks are exacting and require close cooperation, the earliest age at which they can be given is usually 5 or 6.

The initial objective is to associate the principal visual direction with the foveal center and to establish centric fixation. This is followed by hand-eye coordination training to obtain and stabilize correct spatial localization.

The final phase stresses improvement in acuity by training to break down central inhibition and to improve form recognition. Following the attainment of centric fixation and improved acuity, if strabismus is present, work commences to establish binocular fixation and sensory fusion.

Cüppers' method is centered about two instruments which he designed, the Euthyscope (21) and the Coordinator (21).

THE EUTHYSCOPE

This instrument is a modified ophthalmoscope capable of high light intensity. In addition to the customary focusing lenses, it is equipped with a Polaroid filter and a special horizontal rotating disk, housing an open aperture, a dark green filter, and two clear targets, each of the last having a black opaque dot at its center, one dot subtending an angle of 3 degrees at the nodal point of the subject's eye and the other 5 degrees. The angular size of the fundus area illuminated may be set for 7 or 30 degrees.

The Euthyscope is used to create an afterimage for the purposes of teaching centric fixation and enhancing cortical receptivity of foveal impulses. A mydriatic is recommended to provide greater ease in viewing the fundus and in positioning the shadow of the opaque dot over the fovea. Practice in the operation of the instrument is important as it is difficult to use unless one is thoroughly familiar with it.

Training Procedure. The patient is seated in a dimly lit room and directed to fixate a distant target with the eye not receiving treatment.

In strabismus of moderate or high degree, the fixation target should be positioned so that the eye to be treated is centered in the palpebral fissure to allow easy viewing of the fovea. To accomplish this and not have the operator's head block the view of the fixation target, it may be necessary either to position the fixation target to the side of the patient and reflect its image into the fixating eye by means of an adjustable plane mirror (either hand-held or mounted on a stand) or to have the target viewed through a hand-held prism (base out in esotropia and base in in exotropia) to cause a version movement in the desired direction.

Preferably, the patient's head should be secured in a chin and head-rest, especially by a head mount attached to a narrow table. This will ensure no head movement during exposure to the Euthyscope and will also enable the operator to rest his elbow on the table top to steady the hand holding the instrument. An adjustable fixation target attached to the headrest (as those used on slit lamps) will simplify the problem of fixation.

The transformer to which the Euthyscope is connected should be set at 4 to 5 volts to present the proper illumination level to the retina. Setting at a higher voltage to provide more intense illumination is not recommended because stray light may stimulate the fovea and the changing of the afterimage from a positive to a negative form may be excessively delayed.

Prior to exposing the eye to the light of the Euthyscope, a light source in the room is connected to a timing device, the Electric Interval Controller (Light Interval Regulator, Controlled Flasher, Alternosope, Alternator). This device will cause the room light to flash on and off, the light phase, dark phase, and brightness being preset by three separate controls. The flashing serves to facilitate the perception of the induced afterimage, to prolong its duration, and to promote a reversal from the positive form (a reproduction of the light pattern of the stimulus) to a negative form (a reversal of the light pattern of the stimulus). The flashing light source is positioned to illuminate intermittently a surface onto which the afterimage will be projected; it is turned on after exposure with the Euthyscope. During the initial training, the dark phase of the flash is made longer than the light phase (such as 6 seconds for the dark phase and 2 seconds for the light phase) to encourage the appearance of the negative afterimage. As training progresses, the dark phase is gradually shortened and the light phase lengthened until the light phase becomes longer than the dark phase, this in order to prolong the duration of the negative afterimage.

The nonamblyopic eye is stimulated first, to familiarize the patient with the afterimage effects. Once the afterimage is recognized, is perceived in both positive and negative form, and is centered on a fixation target, the amblyopic eye is exposed and the training begins.

To stimulate the eye with the Euthyscope, the instrument is set for the 30-degree field and the green filter is rotated into position to prevent excessive light from stimulating the macula. The operator then locates and focuses on the fovea (the Polaroid filter is not used at this time as it will obscure the foveolar reflex). Either the 3- or 5-degree cover target is then rotated into position and the shadow of the dot centered on the fovea to shield it from light stimulation (Figure 25). The 3-degree target is used if fixation is central or eccentric by less than 3 degrees. The 5-degree spot is used if the angle of eccentric fixation is 3 degrees or more.

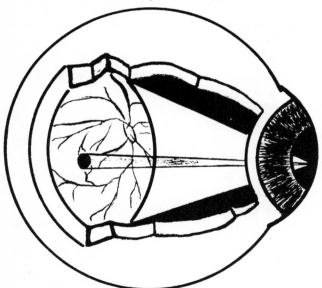

Figure 25. Stimulation of the eye with the Euthyscope to create an afterimage, with the macular area shielded from light stimulation by the shadow cast from a 3-degree or 5-degree opaque target rotated into the light path of the instrument.

Exposure is maintained with the dot target for approximately 25 to 30 seconds. If the exposure is too long, the reversal of the afterimage effect may not occur or may be excessively delayed (the same result occurring if the light intensity is too high). Upon conclusion of the stimulation, the un-exposed eye is occluded, fixation is directed to a silver screen or light-colored wall, and the Electric Interval Controller turned on to produce the preset sequence of intermittent illumination on the fixated surface. The size of the afterimage will vary in direct proportion to the distance of the surface to which it is projected, and its shape will vary in relation to the inclination of this surface.

The positive afterimage is usually perceived first. It resembles the stimulus, appearing as a light circle with a dark center. After a period

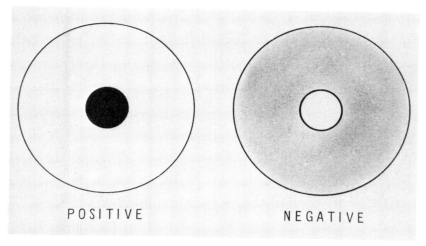

POSITIVE   NEGATIVE

Figure 26. The appearance of the positive and negative afterimage as created by stimulating the eye with the light of the Euthyscope or Projectoscope, the macular area being shielded by the shadow of the opaque dot target.

of time, the negative afterimage will be seen, appearing as a dark circle with a light center (Figure 26). The dark center of the positive afterimage and the light center of the negative afterimage corresponds to the projection from the fovea or macula.

When the negative afterimage is seen, fixation is directed to a form target to determine if the afterimage is centered about it. If eccentric fixation is present, the light center will not be seen centered on the target. If not centered, the patient is instructed to move his eye in the appropriate direction to gain the centering and to hold his eye in this position to maintain it. When achieved, the foveal center will be directed to the target and fixation will be centric. Identification of the form target is attempted once the light center of the negative afterimage is held centered on it. The objective is to reassociate the straight-ahead visual direction with the foveal center and to increase foveal sensitivity.

The afterimage may be induced with a Flash Euthyscope, which is a Euthyscope equipped with a flash mechanism. Once the shadow of the opaque dot is centered on the macula, a button on the instrument's handle is depressed, producing a momentary flash of light of high intensity. A foot switch may be used with the standard Euthyscope to increase automatically the voltage of the transformer to 7½. This enables the operator to locate and focus on the fovea with a low voltage setting and with the dot target in place. Activation of the switch causes a sudden increase in illumination which continues as long as the foot switch is depressed.

The Neitz Euthyscope (20) is patterned after the original Euthyscope by Oculus and may be used in its place. This simple-to-operate ophthalmoscope contains among its special targets a 2- and a 4-degree opaque cover target, each of which is exposed in a 22-degree illuminated field. A flash booster attachment controlled by a hand-held switch is also available.

The Projectoscope with the Nutt Auto-disc attachment also may be used in place of the Euthyscope. The procedure is the same as that used in the Bangerter technique with the exception that the stimulation is completed after the second graticule (which has the 3-degree opaque spot) has been rotated into position and the accompanying intense light exposure has terminated.

Significance of the Afterimages. The afterimages serve not only as a clue to the centricity of fixation and to visual directionalization but also to break down central suppression. They are thus effective in breaking down eccentric fixation and in improving visual acuity when fixation is centric. According to Cüppers, the central retina is inhibited during the positive afterimage, at which time the peripheral retina is dominant. During the negative afterimage, the reverse is considered true; the central retina becomes dominant and central inhibition ceases. Therefore, difficulty may be encountered in obtaining the negative afterimage if central suppression is intense, and several training sessions may be necessary before it is finally perceived.

After continued training, the negative afterimage is perceived more readily and also persists for a longer period of time. The duration of the light and dark phase of the light flash is set with this in mind. The negative afterimage is easier to obtain if the dark phase is longer than the light phase, but it tends to appear during the light phase (against a light background).

The afterimages will eventually fade and should then be restored by repeating the stimulation with the Euthyscope (or Projectoscope). The life of the afterimages may be as long as 20 minutes, tending to increase with experience. Blinking or massaging the eye, in addition to the flashing of light, will prolong their existence.

Fixation of a form target cannot be performed during the presence of the positive afterimage as it is obscured by the black central area of the afterimage. Only when the negative afterimage is present, with its light center, is the target visible. Thus the training cannot proceed unless the negative afterimage can be perceived, and, as the afterimage alternates between the positive and negative form, the training takes place only when the negative form is present.

Monocular Diplopia. Before the straight ahead visual direction becomes reassociated with only the foveal center, an intermediate stage may occur in which the straight-ahead visual direction is simultaneously associated with the site of eccentric fixation and the foveal center. Monocular diplopia will result, as a target stimulating the foveal center will be simultaneously directionalized to two different locations, one location corresponding to the straight ahead direction and the other to the anomalous visual direction which the foveal center has previously demonstrated. Reinforcement of the association of the straight ahead direction with the foveal center will eliminate the anomalous localization and the monocular diplopia.

Fixation Distance. In the early phases of the training, the surface onto which the afterimage is projected is close to the eye (3 to 6 feet). Fixation distance is gradually increased to 20 feet as training progresses, requiring the projection of the afterimage to greater and greater distances.

Fixation Targets. Fixation targets are relatively large at the start and commensurate with the patient's acuity. Identification of the target's form is of secondary importance if eccentric fixation is present. The primary objective is to teach the association of the straight ahead direction with the foveal center; that is, the centering of the negative afterimage around the fixated target. When fixation is centric, both the centering of the negative afterimage around the target and its identification are important, as improvement in form recognition is now stressed.

Routine test type, such as Landolt Cs or Snellen Es, may be used for this training. A novel target employed by Priestley (1960) is a rotating kaleidoscopic pattern (Figure 27). The constantly varying

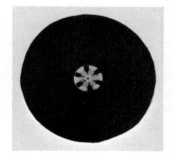

Figure 27. A kaleidoscopic pattern as seen when a negative afterimage is centered on it. (*Reprinted from* International Ophthalmology Clinics, *Vol. 1, No. 4, 1961, by permission of Little, Brown and Co.*)

symmetrical design will stimulate interest and attention and is ideally suited for superimposing and centering the negative afterimage.

Initially the targets are stationary, but, as skill is achieved in the centering of the negative afterimage, movement may be introduced to provide a dynamic and more challenging demand. A means of providing target movement suggested by Priestley (1960) is to present, on one side of a screen, a single Snellen E mounted on the face of a rotatable disk, the disk being controlled by a magnet held against the opposite side of the screen. The target is moved about the screen and the patient required to maintain the centering of the negative afterimage and to identify the orientation of the E.

THE COORDINATOR

Training is given with the Coordinator after fixation has improved from treatment with the Euthyscope and the eccentricity has been reduced or centricity demonstrated, even though it may be inconstant or unsteady, or if fixation is originally centric. The Coordinator is a small table-mounted instrument which produces the entoptic phenomenon of Haidinger's brushes by the transillumination of a target through a rotating Polaroid filter. The target is monocularly viewed through a blue filter which is best suited to produce the brush effect.

The aim of training with the Coordinator is to reinforce centric fixation and to teach hand-eye coordination; that is, to correlate visual directionalization with tactile localization. Haidinger's brushes, which are derived from macular stimulation, are projected into space in relation to a fixation target at a distance of approximately 13 to 16 inches. The fixating eye is voluntarily rotated, if necessary, so that the center of the rotating brushes (produced by the rotating Polaroid filter) is centered on a fixation target, indicating centric fixation. While maintaining this response, the patient positions a pointer held by the patient positioned with its tip in front of the exposed eye, aligned with the fixation target, and then moves to contact it. A correct response is the unhesitating movement of the pointer tip straight to the target while the Haidinger's brushes remain centered on it.

A visuomotor incoordination will be manifested if fixation is eccentric. This is indicated by the need to make a voluntary eye movement to center the brushes on the target, by the failure to identify correctly the physical location of the target with the pointer (anomalous spatial localization), or by the inability to perceive the pointer tip, brushes, and fixation target all at the same locus in space. When the foveal center regains the zero retinomotor value and the principal visual direction, these anomalous responses will no longer occur.

The instrument has controls for varying the illumination of the target and for varying the speed and direction of rotation of the Polaroid filter. A flashing light attachment, mounted externally to the target, may also be used to preserve an afterimage if both the afterimage and the brushes are to be centered on the fixation target.

The rotating Polaroid filter not only makes it easier to observe the brushes by producing a rotating propeller effect but also prevents local adaptation of the retinal receptors. The reversal of the rotation of the Polaroid filter helps to verify the patient's response because a change in the direction of the rotation of the brushes should be reported (clockwise vs. counterclockwise). A reversal of the rotation of the brushes may also be induced by interposing a mounted sheet of clear cellophane between the eye and the target.

The training is performed first with the nonamblyopic eye to familiarize the patient with the brush effect and the localization demands. The room illumination should be dim to aid in the observation of the brushes. The target lighting and the speed of rotation of the Polaroid filter also have a bearing on the ease in which the brushes may be perceived and should be adjusted accordingly.

The brushes may be seen even if vision is considerably reduced (Sherman and Priestley, 1962) but may go unnoticed if fixation is eccentric in excess of 5 to 7 degrees.

As in working with any entoptic phenomenon, the patient must cooperate, have insight and be an astute observer. This training frequently cannot be performed on patients younger than 6 or 7; they cannot be made to understand what it is they are to see and cannot be taught to perform the eye movements necessary to keep the brushes centered on the target.

The target used with the Coordinator is a line drawing of the front view of an airplane. The rotating brushes are to be directed to and centered on the airplane's nose while the pointer is moved to touch this location. A simpler task may be introduced by requiring the patient to fixate and center the brushes on a pointer held by the operator, and to keep the brushes centered on the pointer as it is moved to different areas of the airplane target.

The training may also be performed with the negative afterimage as induced with the Euthyscope. Both the clear center of the negative afterimage and the Haidinger's brushes must now be centered on the fixation target. Circular apertures of successively smaller diameters may be used to limit the field of vision. As the field of vision is progressively reduced, fixation must be more accurate to see the brushes in the smaller field and to keep them centered in the opening.

THE MACULA INTEGRITY TESTER-TRAINER

An instrument that can be used in place of the Coordinator is the Macula Integrity Tester-Trainer. Like the Coordinator, it is a small, table-mounted instrument housing a light source and a motor-driven Polaroid filter. Light is directed through the rotating Polaroid filter to transilluminate an external target mounted on one of its vertical faces. The target is monocularly viewed through a deep blue filter placed either in front of the eye or in front of the target. The rotation of the Polaroid filter may be reversed by interposing a clear cellophane slide (supplied with the instrument) between the eye and the target.

The training procedure is identical to that described for the Coordinator, but the target used is either a clear glass slide or a glass slide containing randomly located black letters of varying size. The letters serve as fixation targets about which the brushes are to be centered. The clear glass slide is used with a pointer which is moved about its surface. The patient attempts to keep the brushes centered on the tip by making the correct eye movement. Apertures of various sizes and configurations placed over the clear glass slide may be made to vary the difficulty of the task and to provide a greater variety of training demands. Spiral-shaped apertures of varying width and length, or a series of two or three circular apertures of varying diameter cut from a single piece of opaque material, are examples of improvised ways to present a greater array of tasks. When using the spiral aperture, the patient is instructed to move his eye along the path of the spiral and to try to keep the center of the rotating brushes always in view and centered in the opening. When using a series of circular apertures, the patient is instructed to change fixation abruptly from the largest circular aperture to a smaller aperture, and to center the brushes each time fixation is changed. Since these dynamic small-field demands are more difficult, they are introduced only after it has been demonstrated that the brushes can be centered on a single fixation target situated in a large field.

THE SPACE COORDINATOR

An extension of the training with the Coordinator is accomplished with the Space Coordinator (21). This instrument also is designed to create the Haidinger's brushes effect, but in this instance both the brushes and the fixation targets are to be projected into space to a screen about 6 feet away. This small, cylindrically shaped apparatus contains a motor-driven Polaroid filter, a deep blue filter, and a light source. At one end is an eyepiece to focus enclosed fixation targets, while the other end is open. It has a diaphragm adjustment for varying the size of an aperture, controls for regulating the speed and direction of rotation of the Polaroid filter, a second supplementary blue filter that can be moved into the field to make the brushes more distinct, and a disk containing four apertures of different diameters to set the maximum field of view. Two ratcheted bar slides are used with the instrument, each containing a series of vertically aligned test targets. The slides are inserted in a slit at the underside of the instrument and adjusted upward, through the top of the instrument, to expose the desired target content in the aperture.

The Space Coordinator is mounted on a tripod situated in front of a reflecting screen and is connected to the same Electric Interval Controller used with the Euthyscope to control the intensity and flashing sequence of its light sources.

Background illumination for the target and brushes is provided by a 500-watt projector, which is directed toward the reflecting screen and angled so that its light is reflected from the screen directly into the open end of the instrument. The untreated eye, instead of being occluded, may be stimulated with blue light derived from a blue filter mounted on a laterally extending rotatable arm attached to the end at which the eyepiece is located. This blue filter is illuminated by a diffuse white light source mounted on a laterally extending rotatable arm attached to the opposite end.

The patient, seated before the instrument, looks through the eyepiece with the amblyopic eye to observe the brushes, the fixation target, and the distant illuminated screen, while the untreated eye remains open and is exposed to blue light created by a transilluminated blue filter positioned in front of it.

Training may be conducted with the brushes alone, with the afterimage created by stimulation with the Euthyscope alone, or with both, with or without a fixation target. If eccentric fixation is present, its magnitude must be less than 5 degrees; otherwise the fovea will be out of the instrument's field of view.

The simplest training offers only the rotating brushes, which are to be directionalized straight ahead to the distant screen. Initially, this may require a voluntary eye movement if fixation is still eccentric, but eventually it should be possible to directionalize the brushes correctly when the patient has the impression that he is looking straight ahead.

Next, the negative afterimage is combined with the brushes. The light source of the instrument may be set to a flash sequence to enhance the afterimage effect. At first only the negative afterimage is directionalized straight ahead to the screen. Once this is achieved, the patient is exposed to the brushes, which are rotating at a speed at which they are most visible. He simultaneously attempts to directionalize the negative afterimage and the brushes straight ahead and to see the rotating brushes in the clear center of the negative afterimage. Repetition and practice may be required; difficulty may be experienced in perceiving the brushes straight ahead and in the center of the negative afterimage. The tendency is to be able to directionalize the negative afterimage straight ahead but to perceive the brushes displaced to the side.

When both the negative afterimage and brushes can be localized correctly straight ahead, fixation is directed to single E targets introduced with the bar slides. At this stage, the brushes should be observed centered on the fixation target without the need of voluntary corrective eye movements. Both the brushes and the fixation target should be projected straight ahead to the surface of the screen. When this has been satisfactorily performed, successively smaller E targets are presented; each time the orientation of the letter is to be identified as it is fixated and seen straight ahead with the brushes centered on it. The task is then made more difficult by adjusting the diaphragm control gradually to reduce the size of the aperture to include just the target.

The final phase of training with the Space Coordinator calls for the introduction of several Es arranged either in a horizontal or vertical row. The aperture is reduced in size to present a single target which is fixated and, together with the brushes, is directionalized straight ahead. The aperture is then slowly increased to expose the neighboring targets while fixation and the brushes continue to be directed to the same letter. When fixation control can be maintained in this fashion, the aperture size is held open, exposing all letters. Fixation is then shifted in turn to each E in the row whose orientation is to be identified as the brushes are centered on it. Progressively smaller targets are used as acuity improves.

A binocular demand may be presented, requiring coordination of the principal visual direction of each eye, by creating an afterimage in the nonamblyopic eye and presenting the brushes to the amblyopic eye. The desired binocular percept is that of the negative afterimage projected straight ahead with the Haidinger's brushes rotating in its clear center. This is in effect training to establish or reinforce normal retinal correspondence.

SYNOPTOPHORE

Training to project the Haidinger's brushes correctly in reference to a fixation target may also be performed on synoptophores (6, 21) specially equipped with attachments to create the brush effect. As with the Space Coordinator, the speed and direction of rotation of the Polaroid filter may be controlled, and an adjustable diaphragm permits a variation in the size of the field. If desired, rotating brushes may be presented simultaneously to the two eyes; if presented to one eye, the other is exposed to a blank, transilluminated blue field.

The Haidinger's brushes unit supplied with the Clement Clarke synoptophore may be used by itself, while electrically connected to the synoptophore, by fixing it to a supplied table mounting having an attached chin rest. It may also be obtained as a separate unit, having its own controls for varying aperture size and speed and direction of rotation of the Polaroid filter (Clement Clark Space Coordinator, Figure 28). Used in this manner, the brushes may be projected into real space to any fixation distance desired. The fixation targets must be located in the plane to which the brushes are projected, since the synoptophore targets cannot now be used.

Shipley (1963) has improvised a battery-operated attachment for the Troposcope (1) to produce the Haidinger's brushes. A small motor drives a pulley to rotate a ball-bearing-mounted disk containing a Polaroid filter and a blue filter (Wratten No. 48A). The disk, which rotates between 10 and 20 rpm, is placed in one of the target slots and may be used in conjunction with the standard targets supplied with this instrument.

Home Training. Some of Cüppers' methods may be performed at home if fixation is centric, even though unsteady or inconstant. This may prove useful in speeding improvement, since Cüppers' technique (and Bangerter's) relies on concentrated daily training.

The afterimage may be produced by placing a black opaque circle approximately 4 cm in diameter with a 3-mm transparent red fixation dot at its center (Priestley, Hermann and Nutter, 1963) onto a 60-

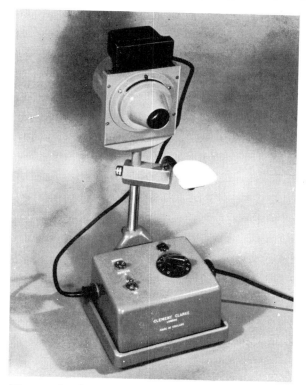

Figure 28. The Clement Clarke Space Coordinator.

watt frosted light bulb. The lighted bulb is exposed to the amblyopic eye for one minute while fixation is maintained on the transparent red dot. The distance of fixation determines the angular size of the retinal area shaded by the black circle (tangent of angular area shielded is equal to 0.04 divided by the fixation distance in meters). At a 46-cm fixation distance, it shields a 5-degree area.

To enhance and prolong the afterimage, the room light may be flashed by plugging it into an inexpensive electric device of the type used for flashing Christmas tree lights. A flash rate of 15 or 100 flashes per minute may be obtained.

The afterimage should be projected onto a light-colored wall on which is secured a fixation target. The negative afterimage is then directed to and centered about this target. With improvement, the fixation distance is gradually increased and the target size reduced.

Training at home with the Haidinger's brushes may be performed on the same instruments used in the office, that is, the Coordinator or the Macula Integrity Tester-Trainer. Rotating Haidinger's brushes may also be produced by the Rinaldi-Larson Dynascope (10), a hand-held battery-operated device designed primarily for home training. Brushes produced with this instrument may be projected onto distant as well as near targets.

Before training is prescribed for home practice, there should be no doubt in the patient's and parents' minds as to the exact procedures to follow and its importance.

Both the patient and the parents should not only be taught the procedures but also should be asked to perform or demonstrate them in the office. Hurriedly prescribed home training will most probably be performed incorrectly or not at all.

The training at home should be for 30-minute periods at least twice a day. At frequent intervals, checks should be made to evaluate progress. Fixation should be retested, as with the Visuscope, and the response compared with that previously recorded. Visual acuity should be remeasured in the same manner originally employed, retesting both single letter acuity and line acuity.

EVALUATION OF BANGERTER'S AND CÜPPERS' METHODS

Following the introduction of their techniques, Bangerter (1955) and Cüppers (1956, 1961) published favorable statistical reports on improvement in visual acuity and fixation which they obtained on patients treated with their respective methods. There subsequently appeared reports by many others which, though differing in statistical results, confirmed the usefulness of these techniques (Clerici and Legorini, 1955; Sevrin, 1956; Thomas and Bretagne, 1956; Belostotsky and Friedman, 1957; de Laet and Szucs, 1956, with Leblois, 1958; Mayweg and Massie, 1958; Capobianco, 1960; Görtz, 1960; Byron, 1960; Girard et al., 1962).

Other reports, however, were critical and voiced dissatisfaction. Some believed that simple occlusion and routine exercises provided essentially the same results as the more complex and elaborate pleoptic procedures (Chinaglia and Andreani, 1955; Gale, 1957). Others felt the techniques were time consuming, inconvenient, and expensive

(Jonkers, 1956; Gale, 1957; Byron, 1960) and so demanding of patience and cooperation that they usually could not be effectively performed on patients younger than 8 to 10 (Lang, 1956; Barraquer, Ariza and Reinoso, 1958). Jonkers (1956, 1959) found the Cüppers technique ineffective if eccentric fixation was stable, and also he was rarely able to achieve normal acuity. Although the pleoptic techniques were effective in breaking down eccentric fixation and restoring centric fixation, von Noorden (1964) found the acuity improvements unimpressive. None of the 58 cases in his study attained normal line acuity, most ending with 20/50 or worse. Von Noorden suggested that line acuity be used as the criterion for acuity improvement rather than single letter acuity; if it were, some of the reported acuity improvements would be less encouraging.

Priestley, Byron and Weseley (1959) mention the multitude of instruments required for the Bangerter technique. Sarrazin (1956) and Barraquer et al. (1958) point out the difficulty of keeping the macula shielded when using the Euthyscope, and von Noorden (1964) mentions the difficulty in maintaining the child's interest with the afterimages involved in the Cüppers approach.

The pros and cons of inverse occlusion have been discussed in Chapter 17; interestingly, Byron (1960) reports better results when occlusion of the fixating eye was not carried out prior to the treatment.

It should be anticipated that the conclusions reached and opinions expressed would run from wholehearted acceptance to rejection. The differences may be attributed partly to the many obvious and subtle variables which could influence the results. The more obvious variables include patient's present age, age of onset, type of fixation, extent of acuity reduction, binocular status, refractive error, methods of classifying the conditions, and statistical treatment of the data. The more subtle variables include frequency of training, duration of training, skill in administering training, how closely and accurately the recommended training procedures were followed, patient and parent intelligence, cooperation and motivation, and attitude and enthusiasm of those conducting the training. These latter variables hold the key to success or failure, not only to the Cüppers or Bangerter methods, but to any training program. Considering all of these variables, it is most difficult to correlate the results of the many studies.

Unquestionably, training is time-consuming, expensive, and demanding, it requires intelligence and cooperation, and it necessitates specialized instrumentation. This is true of visual training in general and is not peculiar to one technique. The Bangerter and Cüppers methods have contributed significantly to the techniques available in treating amblyopia ex anopsia. These techniques should be taken in proper perspective, however, for they represent additional approaches to the treatment of this condition, not techniques that are necessarily intended to supplant or replace previously existing training procedures. Nor should one feel obliged to accept or practice only one method and not the other. Both techniques have merit and can be simultaneously employed to advantage on the same patient.

Perhaps the greatest value of the Bangerter and Cüppers methods is that they offer a means of specifically treating eccentric fixation. Previously used training techniques did not offer sufficient controls on fixation and did not directly train to break down eccentric fixation. Of the two, the Cüppers technique is superior in this respect because centric fixation is forced through the use of afterimages and Haidinger's brushes, and its absence or presence is always detectable.

Of the various types of eccentric fixation, the most resistent to acuity and fixation improvement are the peripheral and the steady, small-angle types. About equally good success in fixation and acuity improvement is obtained in unsteady centric, parafoveal, and paramacular fixation (Wheeler, 1956; Douthwaite and Lee, 1958; Barraquer, Ariza and Reinoso, 1958; Priestley, Byron and Weseley, 1959; Cüppers, 1961; Wild, 1961; von Noorden, 1964).

Both Bangerter and Cüppers stress hand-eye coordination, but the problem of anomalous spatial localization is more effectively dealt with by the Cüppers method, which emphasizes the association of the principal visual direction with the foveal center and the correlation of this principal direction with kinesthetic localization.

The age group which responds most favorably to Cüppers' and Bangerter's methods is generally agreed to be that between 7 and 15, although some include 5- and 6-year-olds (Gale, 1957; Mayweg and Massie, 1958; Barraquer et al., 1958; Byron, 1960; von Noorden, 1964). The younger ages present the greatest potential opportunity for improvement, as the anomalies are not as firmly entrenched and normal functioning is more easily attained, but a lack of cooperation and motivation in these children may negate this advantage.

Smith's Techniques

A variety of training procedures have been devised by William S. Smith (1950, 1954), one of the pioneers in the field of visual training. His recommendations represent one of the first organized approaches for the treatment of the various deficiencies found in amblyopia ex anopsia.

LIGHT STIMULATION

Light stimulation is a preliminary form of training in which the amblyopic eye is exposed to a bright flashing light. The purpose is to stimulate the simple fixation reflex and exercise the synaptic relay of impulses in the visual pathway, thereby countering the effects of disuse or the inhibition influences of suppression. It is given to all amblyopes but especially to amblyopes of long standing and to those manifesting severe reductions in visual acuity.

The procedure is to expose the amblyopic eye to a bright flashing light, as may be provided by many of the standard orthoptic devices, or by a 15-watt frosted bulb mounted in a reflector and connected to an electric flasher unit. No diffusers or targets are used, and either the instrument shields the eye from the external room light to provide a dark chamber or the room lights are dimmed or turned off.

Each treatment lasts 5 to 10 minutes. Training is continued until the patient complains of glare or the eye tears, either reaction indicating that sensitivity has been sufficiently increased to add other training tasks.

TRACING EXERCISES

A special paper tracing plate, devised by Smith, is used for this procedure (Figure 29). The plate contains an array of black line drawings of objects familiar to children, randomly placed and of varying complexity. The pictures are drawn in reverse as the tracing is made on the opposite side of the sheet. The tracing plate is placed face down against a diffusing glass surface (as that of the Omni-

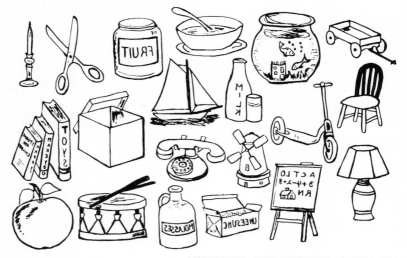

TARGET FOR TRACING — DEVISED BY WILLIAM SMITH, O.D., BOSTON, MASS.

Figure 29. The Smith Tracing Plate.

trainer) and is intermittently transilluminated by a flashing light source situated behind the diffusing glass. The patient, wearing his spectacle correction and with the nonamblyopic eye occluded, is required to trace steadily and accurately over the lines of the selected picture during the periods it is illuminated. Special attention is paid to head posture, care being taken that the head is continually held straight and that no head turning or tilting occurs. The tracing plate is obtainable in pad form (3) and may be used either in the office or for home training.

The purpose of this training procedure is to reinforce the transmission of retinal impulses, teach correct visual projection, and coordinate visual projection with kinesthetic localization.

PROJECTION TRAINING

Training to establish centric fixation and normal spatial localization is also performed with the Smith projection plate described in Chapter 13. The plate consists of a variety of colored drawings, each containing a number of small holes in its interior and at its periphery. With the nonamblyopic eye occluded and the corrective prescription worn, the patient attempts to insert a colored toothpick directly into each of the holes as they are fixated in turn. The toothpick, held at the tip in front of the amblyopic eye, is aimed at a specific opening and then moved rapidly to it. If spatial localization is correct, the toothpick will follow a straight path from the fixating eye to the hole. If spatial localization is anomalous, the toothpick will miss the hole, touch the plate instead, and groping or searching movements will follow in an attempt to locate the opening. If the patient is allowed to move the toothpick slowly to the fixated hole, it will follow a curved path, a corrective movement being made when it is realized that the pick is incorrectly aimed.

Once the picks have been inserted into all the holes of a given picture, an attempt is made to remove them, one at a time, by fixating the protruding tip of each pick and moving the hand from the eye direct to the tip without touching the neighboring picks.

The plate is well illuminated by room light and positioned at a near distance at eye level. The head should be held straight, not tilted or turned. The procedure is performed until accuracy in spatial localization is consistently demonstrated. This plate, like the tracing plate, is available in pad form (3) and may be used in the office or at home.

VISUAL ORIENTATION TRAINING

Visual orientation training is the name given by Smith for training form recognition and the orientation or location in space of a form surrounded by other forms.

Two stereograms have been designed for this purpose. One contains a number of closely grouped, variably sized pictures of familiar objects, and the other contains numerous closely grouped, variably sized numbers and letters (Figure 30).

The stereograms are viewed in a Brewster type stereoscope (as a Telebinocular or Omnitrainer) and are positioned at the optical infinity setting unless the acuity is so reduced as to require a nearer setting. With the spectacle correction worn and the nonamblyopic eye occluded, the patient is asked to fixate each form, identify it, and trace over it with a pointer held in the customarily used hand. Illumination may be constant or intermittent.

This procedure may be considered as a method of attacking the accentuated crowding phenomenon found in strabismic and anisome-

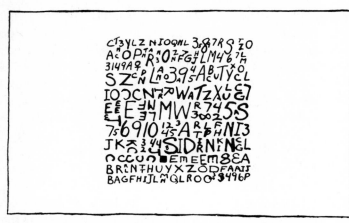

Figure 30. Smith's Visual Orientation Stereogram. (*From Smith:* Clinical Orthoptic Procedure, 2nd ed., St. Louis, 1954, the C. V. Mosby Co.)

tropic amblyopia and may be performed on any similarly constructed stereogram.

VISUAL ACUITY TRAINING

Training to improve visual acuity is performed with a variety of procedures and targets, ranging from identification of letters on an acuity chart to training with stereograms designed by Smith.

The Smith acuity targets consist of a series of split stereograms. Some contain a group of pictures of variable size, some contain variously sized letters, numbers and pictures, and some contain words, gradually decreasing in size, which relate a message.

The target used is commensurate with the patient's corrected acuity and literacy. The stereogram is viewed monocularly in a stereoscope with constant or intermittent illumination. The starting target setting is optical infinity. If difficulty is encountered, the target is moved slowly toward the near setting until identification can be made with certainty. The stereogram is then moved slowly back toward the infinity setting, an attempt being made to continue to identify all of the targets correctly as the infinity setting is reached. Once easy identification is possible at the infinity setting, the stereogram with next smaller target content is used and the procedure is repeated.

If the target carrier is open, the patient is asked to point to and trace over each target as it is fixated and identified. If a flash sequence is employed, the on and off phases are of relatively long and equal duration at the commencement of the training. As progress is made, the rapidity of the cycle is increased, and the sequence is changed so that the off phase is lengthened and the on phase is decreased.

Many commercially available stereograms with appropriate form content may be used in the same manner.

ACCOMMODATION TRAINING

Smith has noted that the amblyopic eye demonstrates a lower amplitude of accommodation than the fellow eye and an impaired ability to alter accommodation in response to abruptly presented changes in dioptric demand. The same observation was made by Abraham (1961), who found that even after the amblyopic eye attained normal acuity it continued to demonstrate a weakened ability to meet changes in accommodative demand at far and near and a lower amplitude of accommodation than the fellow eye. Abraham attributes the weakened accommodative ability in anisometropic and strabismic amblyopia to the disuse of the amblyopic eye in initiating the accommodative reflex.

Crane's report (1966) on the factors initiating and controlling the accommodative response provides other possible reasons why an amblyopic eye exhibits poor accommodative facility. He points out that the focus control of the eye operates on signals received from only a small central portion of the fovea, approximately 30 seconds in diameter.

If eccentric fixation is present, or if this small central area is reduced in sensitivity due to inhibition, or if fixation is unsteady or jerky, this central foveal area could not function normally in response to an out-of-focus retinal image. The image of the fixed target would either not stimulate this area (eccentric fixation), would not induce a precise accommodative response (reduced sensitivity), or, by constantly moving about the central area, would cause variations in the signals.

Training for accommodative facility in amblyopia ex anopsia may be performed with a stereoscope by alternately presenting different dioptric demands to the eyes. The stereogram used should contain a variety of fixation targets of appropriate size, and a flash sequence should be used to illuminate alternately the material presented to each eye. The time permitted for fixating and clearing is gradually reduced as improvement takes place. The accommodative demands may be varied by placing concave or convex lenses in the cells of the instrument, the dioptric powers and the difference between them being commensurate with the patient's ability.

Accommodative flexibility training may also be given by having the patient quickly (and alternately) shift monocular fixation back and forth between distant and near targets. The fixation distances selected will determine the dioptric demands, and these demands may be altered by placing lenses of various dioptric power before the eye or eyes.

In addition to the procedure he originated, Smith has adapted procedures devised by others to his own purposes and incorporated them into his organized program. He continually stresses the need for persistent repetition of a training task to achieve results. He recognizes the desirability of administering the training as frequently as possible and emphasizes the importance of having the training supervised by one who is not only skilled and experienced but also determined and tenacious.

Otwell's Technique

A training approach devised by Harry C. Otwell (1958) for the treatment of amblyopia ex anopsia and strabismus, called Therapeutic Orthoptics, is claimed to enjoy rather spectacular results. Otwell states that his treatment for amblyopia ex anopsia will restore acuity in a high percentage of the cases to 20/50 or better within a few days, even in older patients, and has published many case findings reporting such results (1960, 1963, 1965, 1966).

Two instruments are used for amblyopia treatment, both devised by Otwell, one the Sodium Light Flash unit is primarily for home training and the other the Electronic Orthoptor for office training.

The Sodium Light Flash Unit. This device consists of a flashing light source and a unit composed of a pinhole disk, a condensing lens, and an amber (sodium) filter. The flashing light is positioned about 8 inches from the eye and is viewed monocularly for approximately 12 minutes through the correcting lens and the pinhole unit. Immediately following this stimulation, and with the nontreated eye occluded, the resulting afterimage is projected onto a light-colored vertical surface approximately 10 feet distant. The size of the afterimage is then observed. According to Otwell, its diameter may be very small, but as inhibition influences are broken down, it will gradually increase in size to approximately 10 inches.

The Electronic Orthoptor. The Electronic Orthoptor is a stereoscopic device equipped with a standard stereoscopic head (+5.00 diopter base out, spheroprism eyepieces, optical center separation 95 mm), pinhole disks, and two rotating disks, one before each eye, containing a red filter, an amber filter, and two open apertures. A built-in, preset electric timer provides an alternating flash of 144 cycles per minute, or 4 seconds on and 1.5 seconds off, to each eye individually or to both eyes synchronously. The light source separation may be varied laterally to meet the requirements of binocular stimulation, and a target support enables the use of standard stereograms.

In amblyopia treatment with the Electronic Orthoptor the amblyopic eye views the flashing light through the lens correction and the pinhole disk and amber filter for a period of 12 minutes. The flash cycle is set for 4 seconds on and 1.5 seconds off. Immediately following this stimulation, the treatment continues with the projection of the afterimage, as described for the home training unit.

The treatment is given twice daily, initially at the office and then at home, and is continued as long as acuity improvement occurs. No occlusion is practiced between training sessions, and the procedure followed is the same regardless of the type of fixation. The corrected visual acuity is determined prior to and 20 minutes after treatment.

The purpose of this therapy is to increase the sensitivity of the central retinal receptors. Otwell considers the amber light to be most effective for this stimulation.

When acuity has improved to 20/40 or better, binocular stimulation is presented to treat suppression in strabismus and to establish or improve sensory and motor fusion. The suppression treatment is primarily one of exposing the eyes to the rapid alternating-flash sequence, using the red filters, until two lights are simultaneously observed when both light sources are turned on. Auxiliary prisms are then used, and/or the separation of the light sources is altered, so that the lighted areas may be superimposed and fused. The rapid alternating-flash sequence is designed to create cortical "confusion" and thereby break down the cortical block. (Further details of the procedures are beyond the scope of this text.)

Allen's Method

The technique introduced by Merrill J. Allen (1966) has as its basis the Bartley phenomenon, the perceptual increase in brightness experienced when a surface is intermittently illuminated by a flash sequence at or near the alpha rhythm of the brain, as compared to that experienced with steady illumination of the same intensity. An explanation of this brightness enhancement is that the intermittent light stimuli are of such duration that no time is permitted for the buildup of normal inhibitory interactions.

Allen has applied this knowledge to clinical use by devising instruments suitable for the treatment of visual abnormalities which preclude normal binocular functioning, such as amblyopia, suppression, and anomalous correspondence. To break down these anomalies, light stimulation is presented alternately (or simultaneously) in rapid succession to the two eyes. The alternating flash sequence is timed to set up a train of impulses from the two eyes which arrive at the lateral geniculate body asynchronously.

The intent is to force the normal use of the visual pathway from each eye to the visual cortex by setting up a stimulus condition in which the train of impulses from the two eyes joins to form a continuous flow, the train of impulses from one eye arriving exactly out of phase with those from the other eye. This type of stimulation is intended to bypass the neural defense mechanism of suppression which would occur if the impulses arrived simultaneously or at an alternation rate at which the impulse from one eye was still being processed when the impulse from the other eye arrived. Hence, with this asynchronous method of alternate photic stimulation, binocular reception is approached as closely as possible without inciting suppression or neural inhibition.

THE TRANSLID BINOCULAR INTERACTION TRAINER

To produce such light stimulation, Allen has designed the Translid Binocular Interaction Trainer, or T.B.I. Trainer (24). It is a battery-operated, transistor-controlled dual source of light mounted at the head of a flashlight handle (Figure 31). The instrument provides an alternating flash, stimulating each eye at a rate of 7 to 10 times per second. The light cycle is a square wave having equal dark and light phases.

The training is performed both at home and in the office. The recommended procedure is first to place the flashing light source (separated for the P.D.) gently against the closed upper eyelids for 3 to 5 minutes. Following this stimulation, the eyes are opened and each light source is placed close to and directly in front of the corresponding eye. Each eye is to look at its light bulb, essentially by staring straight ahead as the lights are alternately flashing, for a 3- to 5-minute period. The two bulbs should appear to occupy the

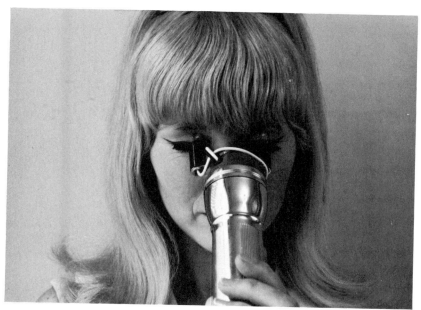

Figure 31. The Translid Binocular Interaction Trainer.

same location when properly adjusted and when binocularity is restored.

The procedures with the eyes closed and then open are repeated for periods of from 10 to 30 minutes, eight times a day, with a minimum rest interval of 30 minutes. It is continued for at least 10 days, and longer if further progress is anticipated.

Between training periods, binasal or total monocular occlusion is practiced to prevent the use of, or need for, suppression. Acuity training through correcting lenses may be given concurrently.

A factor to be considered in prescribing this training is that the intermittent light stimulation of the eyes at the proper frequencies may induce, in susceptible persons, a seizure that resembles an epileptic seizure. Allen, in recognizing this possibility, has set the frequency of the light stimulation below that which would normally induce a photoconvulsive response. As a precautionary measure, however, the stimulation should first be given in the office to determine if any distress symptoms result. If so, the stimulation should be discontinued immediately.

THE ROTATING SECTORED DISK

Another means of providing rapid intermittent stimulation to the eyes is afforded by directing fixation to a target seen through a rotating open-sectored disk. The speed of rotation and the open-sectored spacing determine the frequency and duration of each exposure.

A rotating sectored disk (Fusionaider) has been designed by Allen (24) to create this type of intermittent stimulation (Figure 32). The device is a small, hand-held, electrically operated, open-sectored disk, with sector spacings and speed of rotation designed to provide 7½ exposures per second to each eye alternately (or simultaneously). The frequency of stimulation is below that which will normally induce a photoconvulsive response.

The recommended training procedure is to view familiar moving objects through the rotating open-sectored disk for 10 to 15 minutes every hour. The training may be given along with other training procedures and is continued from 3 days to 3 weeks.

This stimulation is intended to overcome suppression and anomalous correspondence by providing an exposure cycle at which brightness enhancement is nearly maximum.

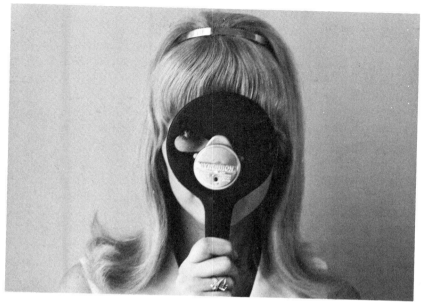

Figure 32. Rotating sectored disk: the right eye momentarily exposed, the left eye momentarily occluded.

The alternation of fixation involved introduces a motor demand which, it is claimed, will in some instances reduce or eliminate a strabismic deviation, although training may not yet have resulted in sensory fusion.

THE PEGBOARD DISK

The Pegboard Disk was designed by Allen to improve pursuit fixation, spatial localization, and eye-hand coordination. The disk is 12 inches in diameter and its surface is striped by 1-inch-wide colored bands, each band containing down its center a series of perforations in linear formation. The disk is attached to a table-mounted motor (Master Rotator) which rotates at a constant speed, either clockwise or counterclockwise. The disk may be orientated in any position from horizontal to vertical. With the nonamblyopic eye occluded, the task is to fill all of the perforations with matching colored golf tees in the shortest possible time for the given plane orientation of the disk. An added task is to place golf balls on the tees when the rotating disk is horizontal without knocking off other golf balls.

As a means of determining progress, a record is made of the time required to fill all the perforations for each position of the disk. This apparatus is also used to train accommodation, stereopsis, convergence, and sensory and motor fusion.

The same training may be performed on a simplified motor (Junior Rotator), which rotates clockwise only.

A small cylinder (Barber Pole), which contains on its surface spirally orientated anaglyphic Landolt Cs or objects familiar to children, may be placed in an opening of the Pegboard Disk to train acuity, fixation, accommodation or convergence as it rotates toward and away from the eyes.

THE AURAL FEEDBACK DISK

This instrument consists of a table-mounted, motor-driven rotating disk having an off-center photosensitive element approximately 6 mm in diameter. The disk is vertically orientated, is colored in sectors whose apexes meet near the disk's periphery, and is driven by either of the motor units used with the Pegboard Disk. The photocell, when activated by a beam of light centered on it, initiates a sound-producing circuit.

Pursuit fixation and spatial localization are trained by requiring the patient to fixate and follow monocularly (or binocularly) the photosensitive element and to direct and maintain the beam of a focusable projecting flashlight on the center of the photocell so that a continuous sound is emitted.

ROTATIONS DISK

The Rotations Disk is similar in design to the Aural Feedback Disk but has a fixation target at the off-center location where the apexes of the colored sectors meet, in place of a photocell. The painted sectors are spaced and colored to provide a 7-cycle-per-second, on-off effect to the peripheral photoreceptors. The disk is driven by the same motor unit used with the Pegboard Disk.

The Groffman Visual Tracing Graphs

An interesting series of exercises has been designed by Sidney Groffman for the treatment of perceptual dysfunctions, reading disabilities, and amblyopia ex anopsia. The purpose of the training is to develop ability in tracing fixation, spatial localization and orientation, and oculomotor coordination. The task is to direct the eye correctly along the path of a continuously winding black line, without the aid of a pointer, and then to trace over this line manually with a colored pencil. The complexity of the task is slowly increased by presenting a longer and more tortuously winding line and by adding additional interweaving lines which must also be traced visually and then tactually.

The starting point of each line is indicated by a capital letter on the left side of the target and the end point by a number on the right side. The patient visually traces over the lines from the starting point to the end point and records, in a space provided at the bottom of each target, the number at which the lines terminate. He then tactually traces over the lines. If the visually determined end point is correct, the manual tracing reinforces the response; if incorrect, the manual tracing will reveal the error. A differently colored pencil is used for each line traced.

Two books of tracing graphs are provided (13). Book 1 contains introductory frames, frames of two, three, and four interweaving stimulus lines of simple and complex discriminations, and five "criterion" frames used to evaluate progress. Book 2 is more difficult and contains frames of four interweaving lines of complex design, frames of three stimulus lines of simple and complex discrimination with five possible responses, frames of five stimulus lines of simple and complex discrimination, and five criterion frames.

The training, as outlined by Groffman, is programmed to permit the patient, after indoctrination, to work at his own pace, with complete independence, so that this learning will be self-instructional. The only time he is to be supervised is when he has progressed to a "criterion" frame. He is then asked to trace visually each line in this frame and state orally at which number it ends. If correct, the training progresses to more complex patterns; if incorrect, it returns to simpler demands unless 75 percent of the teaching frames are correct.

For amblyopia training, the target is either monocularly fixated in a Correct-Eye-Scope (or similar stereoscope which permits tracing), is fixated directly, or is viewed with one eye in a stereoscope and traced with the other (cheiroscopic tracings), assuming normal correspondence. An afterimage created by a Euthyscope or Projectoscope may also be projected along the path of the lines.

The training may be performed in the office or at home for periods of no longer than 15 minutes. Special test frames are used to evaluate the visual tracing performance before and after training.

The Zweig-Bruno Perceptual Development Series

A series of tracing targets has been designed by Richard L. Zweig and Muriel E. Bruno to train hand-eye coordination and direction. Although this training was originated to treat perceptual diffi-

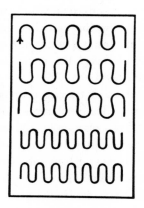

Figure 33. A target in the Zweig-Bruno Perceptual Development Series.

culties associated with reading problems, it does serve as a useful procedure in the treatment of amblyopia ex anopsia.

The targets consist of lines forming various geometric patterns and joined letters (Figure 33). The lines are traced from top to bottom and left to right. The complexity of the targets gradually increases, beginning with straight lines and simple designs and progressing to circles, arcs, curves and letters.

Two pads of these targets are available (13), each pad containing three series of targets in duplicate. As adapted to amblyopia training, the target is viewed monocularly in a stereoscopic instrument which permits tracing (as the Correct-Eye-Scope, Hand-Eye Coordinator, or Stereo-Reader), or is viewed directly. The task is to trace correctly over the line drawing with a colored pencil, and to retrace with a pencil of another color if errors are made. The patterns may also be used for cheiroscopic drawings using the same stereoscopes.

The Leavell Language-Development targets (13) may also be adapted for amblyopia training. These targets consist of line drawings, words, phrases or digits, which may be fixated in a stereoscope and traced, either monocularly or cheiroscopically.

Brock's Techniques

The anaglyph principle has been extensively used by Frederick W. Brock to treat a variety of visual anomalies. Most of the procedures stress binocular fixation, stereopsis, and fusion, but some treat fixation in amblyopia by requiring monocular fixation and localization in the presence of binocular vision. The Brock Posture Board (15), described in Chapter 14, and a simplified version (the MC Trainer) are the primary instruments used for that purpose.

The target content may be black print on a white background or a maze or drawings printed in light red on a white background. If black reading material is placed under the instrument's red filter plate and viewed through complementary colored red and blue-green filters, the print is seen only by the eye viewing through the red filter. The green filter absorbs all the red light, causing the entire red-covered field to appear black. Thus, if the red filter is placed before the amblyopic eye, it alone is exposed to and must interpret the print, although the surrounding visual field is visible to both eyes.

The form targets, printed in light red, are placed on top of the red filter plate while a small white light is directed from below, through the red plate. When this target content is viewed through complementary colored red and blue-green filters, the light red target content is seen as black through the blue-green filter but is invisible through the red filter, the red target content blending in with the red color imparted by the red filter. The light directed through the red plate is seen only with the eye viewing through the red filter, the red imparted to the light being more intense, and standing out, against the lighter red background. The red light cannot be seen through the blue-green filter because the filter absorbs the red wavelength, and the reflection of room light from the white surface of the target through the blue-green filter imparts a green color to this and the surrounding area.

Thus, in the target field, one eye sees only the form content as black while the other eye sees only the red light source. The surrounding field is visible to both eyes. Training is performed by having the amblyopic eye view through the green filter and fixate and follow the maze or form outline while the red light, visible to the other eye, is moved synchronously along the path of fixation.

Other Techniques

TACHISTOSCOPIC TRAINING

The tachistoscope offers an excellent means of training fixation and acuity. A variety of targets is flashed onto a screen for very brief intervals ranging in time from 1/10 of a second to approximately 1/200 of a second. By confining the exposure time to no less than 1/10 of a second, only one fixation is permitted per flash.

The challenge of attempting to identify correctly and/or duplicate the target content for each flash creates intense concentration and continued motivation in both children and adults. Maximum cortical attention is highly conducive to improvement in fixation and visual acuity.

The target content may consist of drawings of familiar objects, geometric forms, digits, words, phrases or sentences. The complexity of the task is increased as progress is made. The instrument especially useful for this purpose is the Keystone Overhead Tachistoscope because of the availability of a large array of targets.

Prior to the training, the patient should be informed of the procedure and directed to fixate a point on the screen about which the stimulus will be centered, and just before each flash he should be alerted by an evenly emphasized "ready—now!" before the shutter release is tripped. A few trial runs should provide familiarization with the demand and target content. In training for amblyopia, the nonamblyopic eye is occluded.

The customary routine is for the patient to record his interpretation of the target after each exposure. The same target is then projected on time exposure to permit a comparison with the recorded response. The response is then scored correct or incorrect and, if incorrect or incomplete, the correct or complete response may then be made. The training is given for approximately 10 or 15 minutes and a record made of the score (number of correct responses over number exposed).

A variation in the use of the tachistoscope is a procedure termed *serial reproduction*. A complex line drawing is flashed onto the screen at a given speed, and the patient is instructed to reproduce the drawing as best he can. This drawing is then concealed and the same form is flashed onto the screen. The patient again draws his interpretation, attempting to correct errors and omissions made in the first drawing. The procedure is repeated about four times, the visual memory of each previous exposure helping to improve each subsequent drawing. The target is then projected on time exposure so that all the detail in the target may be observed and a comparison made with the drawings.

The technique of *form emergence* may also be used with the tachistoscope or any other projecting instrument. A complex form is projected onto a screen so out of focus that it cannot be interpreted. The patient is instructed to fixate and study the blurred image as it is slowly brought into focus and to attempt to identify the form as soon as possible.

DISTANCE MOTIVATION

The technique of distance motivation is intended to improve form identification with visual memory serving as a clue. Acuity targets are monocularly fixated by the amblyopic eye at a distance of approximately 20 feet. The target size should be just below the acuity threshold, such as 20/40 if the acuity is 20/50. The patient slowly walks toward the targets, or the targets are slowly moved toward the patient, until correct identification is possible. The fixation distance is then slowly increased, the attempt being made to reach the starting distance while maintaining correct identification. The visual memory of the previously experienced correct identification assists in the interpretation at the more remote distances.

The procedure is repeated with different targets of the same size. When, eventually, correct identification of targets of this size occurs without the need to reduce fixation distance, the target size is reduced to the next lower Snellen level.

The task may be varied by intermittently illuminating the targets, which may be accomplished by using targets transilluminated with a flashing light source (as performed by Smith) or by connecting the light source in the room to a flasher socket.

The Updegrave Method may be adapted to this type of acuity training. Intermittently illuminated reading material of various size type is presented at near distance and is monocularly fixated by the amblyopic eye. The near distance is adjusted to enable correct identification of the reading material and then gradually increased as the material is being read. When the distance is increased to the point where the print can no longer be correctly interpreted, it is slowly decreased until it can again be read. The distance is then slowly increased once again, the goal being to work to a more remote distance before blurring is noted. Smaller type is used as improvement is made. The reading may be performed through plus or minus lens additions to improve the accommodative response.

The Keystone Reading Series may be similarly used in a stereoscope. These stereograms contain Snellen-rated reading material, some with two sizes of type, an upper paragraph of larger type and a lower paragraph of smaller type. The type size used is dependent upon the level of acuity present.

The stereogram is presented monocularly to the amblyopic eye at the optical infinity setting, and, if necessary, the target holder is slowly moved toward the eyepieces until the print can be read with certainty. As the patient continues to read, the target holder is very slowly edged back toward the infinity setting. When the reading material can be easily read at the infinity position, the procedure is continued with the stereogram in the series having the next smaller type.

If performed on the appropriate stereoscope, the illumination may be varied, the print may be intermittently illuminated, and plus or minus lens additions may be used to include accommodative training.

CHEIROSCOPIC TRAINING

Training to improve fixation, form identification, and break down central suppression are all involved in cheiroscopic training. A stereoscope is used to expose one eye to a line drawing and the other eye to a blank stage on which the image of the target is visually projected and traced. This stimulus condition can be met by any of the stereoscopes that have an accessible stage of sufficient size to receive the projected image. The Leavell Hand-Eye Coordinator, Correct-Eye-Scope, Stereo-Reader, Maddox and Lloyd cheiroscopes (or stereocampimeters), Pigeon-Cantonnet stereoscope, Bernell PSC device, and Tibbs Binocular Trainer are examples of such instruments.

Since one eye sees only the target and the other only the stage and the tracing pencil, binocular vision is necessary if both the target's image and the pencil are to be seen simultaneously. The posture of the fixating eye is controlled by the placement of the target in the instrument and is usually straight ahead. The posture of the eye viewing the blank stage is determined by the direction and magnitude of the phoria or tropia and the influence of proximal convergence.

To be perceived on the projected image, the pencil point must be so located on the platform that its image will fall on a retinal site which corresponds directionally with the retinal site in the fixating eye that receives the target's image. If normal correspondence and centric fixation are present, the image of the fixated target will fall on the fovea of one eye and the image of the pencil point will fall on the fovea of the other eye.

Cheiroscopic drawings should not be prescribed if anomalous correspondence is present since the fovea of one eye corresponds in visual direction with an extrafoveal area of the other eye and cheiroscopic drawings would tend to intensify the anomaly.

The target may be presented to either eye, but contrary to what may be expected more trouble is usually encountered when the amblyopic eye is viewing the blank stage.

The target content is simple at first and gradually increases in complexity as the training progresses. Serial targets may be used in which more and more detail is added to the same picture, in much the same manner as targets used by Bangerter with the Mnemoscope.

To avoid a conflict of crossing borders and the resulting retinal rivalry, the tracing may be made parallel to the projected image, instead of directly on it, or a stylus may be used, the tracing being recorded by carbon paper.

One must be on the alert for signs of suppression when the tracing is made because a good reproduction of the drawing may be made by esotropes even though suppression is present. The pencil point, the tracing and the projected image should all be seen simultaneously, and the only eye movements made should be those involved in following the outline of the target. Disappearance of the tracing, the projected image, or the pencil, or alternations in fixation, are indicative of suppression.

In exotropes, the typical suppression reaction is the constant shifting in location of the projected image on each attempt to place the pencil on it. This is due to an alternation of suppression and fixation. When attention is directed to the pencil to commence the tracing, fixation is shifted straight ahead to the pencil and away from the target. This causes the eye exposed to the target to move templeward from its straight ahead position. The resulting shift in retinal location of the target's image causes it to be projected to another location in space. When fixation is now directed back to the target and away from the pencil, the projected image returns to its original location. Thus, as straight ahead fixation alternates between target and pencil, the projected image continually appears to jump in location and the patient is frustrated in his efforts to trace over it. If this reaction is manifested, it is recommended that cheiroscopic tracings be discontinued, at least temporarily.

PLATEAU'S SPIRAL

Plateau's spiral is a circular white disk on which is painted a black spiral band with its origin at the disk's center. When the disk is rotated and fixation directed to its center, the spiral band gives an illusion of a megaphonelike structure, with its small end extending forward or backward depending on the direction of rotation of the disk. Following exposure to the rotating disk, if fixation is directed to a stationary target, it will appear to swell in size and move forward or shrink in size and recede, the apparent movement being opposite to the perceived megaphone effect.

The apparent movement of the stationary target is considered a motion afterimage effect. The stationary target, by being motionless, is perceived as though it were moving in the opposite direction of the previously experienced stimulation.

The motion afterimage effect induced by exposure to the rotating Plateau's spiral may be applied to fixation and acuity training. If the spiral is fixated with the disk rotating so that the small end of the megaphone effect appears to extend backward, and fixation is then directed to acuity targets, the targets will, for a short time, appear to balloon forward and increase in size. The apparent decrease in distance and increase in target size may serve to enhance identification of form.

The illusion created by the rotating spiral also serves to encourage steady fixation on the spiral's center. Bangerter has applied this pattern in the design of his Centrophor and has further utilized this effect by placing acuity targets at the center of the spiral.

A related effect, also used to improve acuity, is the *waterfall visual illusion*. A motion afterimage is created by viewing a scene designed to give the effect of water, as in a waterfall, continuously flowing in a given direction. Stationary objects, subsequently viewed, will appear to move in the opposite direction of the flowing water.

PERIPHERAL STIMULATION

Stimulation of the peripheral retina is considered by many to provide a relative increase in foveal sensitivity and consequently improved fixation and acuity. This concept is the basis for the peripheral stimulation provided with Bangerter's Pleoptophor and Cüppers' Euthyscope.

In addition to these techniques, peripheral stimulation, prior to acuity training, may be provided by exposing the amblyopic eye to a projected kaleidoscopic pattern or to a rotating disk painted in a pattern of bright colors (as the Aural Feedback Disk on the Arneson Squint Korector).

Another method is afforded by the Renshaw concentric black and green ring slide. This target contains a series of concentric and alternate bands of bright green and black. The slide is projected onto a screen, and the amblyopic eye fixates its center as steadily as possible. After a brief interval of steady fixation, portions of the green rings will suddenly and momentarily turn black. The blotching in of the green rings is attributed to photochemical exhaustion of the retinal receptors and signals the termination of the exposure. An acuity chart is then projected on the screen and an effort made to identify targets smaller than was possible prior to the stimulation.

PURSUIT AND SACCADIC FIXATIONS

In amblyopia ex anopsia, pursuit and saccadic fixations tend to be slow, inaccurate, and erratic. It is therefore desirable that the training program include exercises to improve these fixational movements. Such training, sometimes termed *ocular calisthenics,* is given after steady centric fixation is present.

Monocular pursuit fixations (monocular rotations) may be given by directing fixation to a continuously visible moving target. The speed of movement should be slow enough to enable constant fixation, the movement should be rhythmical, and the extent of the excursion should be well within the limits of the field of fixation.

Many orthoptic instruments feature automatically controlled rotating targets, and some include controls for varying the speed and direction of rotation and the extent of the excursion. Any of such instruments may be used to exercise pursuit fixation, but those which enable easy observation of the eye are more desirable. The strobe light attachment of the Keystone Rotator serves as an ideal fixation target because the light flickers only if fixation is inaccurate.

The fixation distance for directly fixated targets is dependent upon the size of the fixation target, the level of visual acuity, and the extent of the excursion desired. Most typically it ranges between 2 and 5 feet. Each training period is of relatively short duration, approximately 3 to 5 minutes.

Monocular rotations may also be given with manually controlled targets, such as a hand-held penlight. This is useful for home training or to provide a greater versatility in the direction of movement.

Pursuit training is continued until the movement is consistently smooth and accurate and free from any irregularities such as jerkiness or momentary loss of fixation.

Saccadic fixations involve the abrupt shift in fixation from one target to another target. This demand may be introduced in a number of ways and in different degrees of difficulty. The simplest is to present to the one eye a number of stationary targets, each of which is to be fixated in a designated sequence.

A slightly more difficult task is to present to each eye a series of stationary targets which are to be alternately fixated. A yet more difficult task is to present to the one eye an intermittently visible moving target (a combination of pursuit and saccadic fixation). The most difficult task is to present to each eye an intermittently and alternately visible moving target, one eye locating, fixating, and following a target as it appears before one and disappears before the other.

Monocular saccadic fixation of stationary targets may be performed in a stereoscope with stereograms containing a number of fixation targets, or by sequentially fixating a series of targets directly visible. In the latter instance, target forms specifically designed for this purpose are available (as with the Bernell PSC device), or objects in the normal field of vision may serve as fixation targets.

The alternate fixation of stationary targets is performed by employing an alternate flash sequence on a stereoscope, or by alternately fixating targets directly visible on either side of a septum which separates the field of vision of the two eyes. The stereoscope cards designed for this purpose usually have targets placed in opposite directions of the field of gaze, as to the right eye a target up and to the right, and to the left eye a target down and to the left (Smith Fixation Targets, Keystone Specific Muscle Calisthenic Unit).

The Movie Series used with the Keystone Orthotrainer is uniquely constructed to create, when alternately fixated, the illusion of movement based on the phi phenomenon. For example, a monkey is seen hanging by his tail from a tree limb in one position by one eye and in another position with the other eye. With the proper flash sequence, proper positioning of targets (the tree limb alternately stimulating corresponding areas), and prompt alternate fixation, the monkey appears to be swinging back and forth.

An intermittently visible and moving target may be presented to one eye, or alternately to the two eyes, with a stereoscope equipped with both a flash and rotatory mechanism (such as the Rotoscope). Alternately visible and rotating targets may also be introduced manually in conjunction with a hand-held septum positioned at the bridge of the patient's nose. As the target is moved from one side of the septum to the other, the stimulated eye must resume fixation.

The alternate fixation of targets may be performed through auxiliary lenses to produce a different dioptric demand to accommodation to each eye. This arrangement will add to the saccadic fixation demand, training to improve the accuracy and facility of accommodation (accommodative rock training).

If stationary targets are fixated, either by only one eye or alternately, a spatial localization demand may be added by requiring the patient to point to and touch each target as it is fixated.

Saccadic fixation training is practiced until the treated eye can consistently demonstrate a rapid, smooth and precise movement upon shifting fixation from one target to another, whether it be stationary or rotating.

HOME TRAINING

Daily training at home can be an invaluable adjunct to office training and may completely supplant office training for young children. Unquestionably, the rate of improvement will be significantly accelerated, especially in older age groups, if effective stimulation can be given at home, between office visits, instead of a few times a week only at the office.

One must be certain that the home training procedures are carried out properly. The patient (and parents) should practice the procedure in the office so that the steps involved are known, correctly followed, and remembered. Printed instructions alone do not suffice, but they do serve as reminders.

One method of reinforcing a child's memory of a technique is to teach him the technique in the absence of his parents. The child is told that he will be taught how to do an exercise which he will be doing at home and that, after he has learned it, his parents will be called in and he will show them what he is to do. The child usually enjoys the opportunity of being able to demonstrate to his parents what he has been taught, and this challenge acts to promote concentration. During the course of the demonstration to the parents, forgotten points will be reviewed and emphasized, and, at the same time, the parents will be familiarized with the procedure.

Patient and parent motivation and cooperation is an absolute necessity if home training is to be effective. Motivation and cooperation are not automatically forthcoming from children. They must be instilled through the use of psychology and ingenuity. The ability to work with children and induce a desire to cooperate is dependent on intuitive skill in understanding children, in being able to communicate with them at their level, and in establishing a warm rapport.

The child must like the practitioner and be anxious to do as instructed to please him and to qualify for awards given in recognition not only of his accomplishments but, perhaps more important "trying hard." Bringing to the office daily "scores" and "grades" his performance provides information about progress made at home and serves as a constant incentive to receive praise and prizes. Prizes may be awarded each time he "breaks a record" by getting a better score or for getting good grades for trying. Further incentive may be created by putting the child in competition with other children taking training. Posting the names of other patients on a chart, and placing gold stars beside each name, is an example of how this may be done.

If the voluntary cooperation of the child cannot be obtained, despite such efforts, and the child must be coerced by his parents through threats and spankings, home training should be temporarily discontinued. Persisting under such conditions will create emotional disturbances in the child and parents and the training will probably be unproductive even if the child is forced to comply.

Training prescribed for home practice should be uncomplicated and, when possible, entertaining and challenging. The demands should be within the patient's capability, so as not to frustrate or discourage him, but should be difficult enough to require effort and promote improvement. Only a few procedures should be given at one time to avoid confusion; at reasonable intervals, new "games" should replace those already practiced to avoid boredom and monotony. As the simpler tasks are mastered, the difficulty should be increased.

If visual acuity is markedly reduced, it is advisable to confine the training to stationary near-point situations. As acuity improves, the working distance may be increased and movement may be added.

There are many exercises that may be practiced at home. These include the Brinker-Katz red lens occlusion, the Humphriss method, and some of the techniques of Bangerter (as the Centrophor), Cüppers, Smith, Otwell, Allen, Groffman, Zweig-Bruno, and Brock. Other techniques previously mentioned which may also be performed at home are distance motivation, cheiroscopic drawing, accommodative facility training, and pursuit and saccadic fixation training.

In addition, many commercially available games and toys fulfill some of the requirements for amblyopia training and are frequently used for this purpose. Examples are jigsaw puzzles, coloring and tracing books, cutout books, model toys to be constructed or assembled, sewing kits, children's storybooks, stringing colored beads, erector sets, Tinker Toys, marbles and jacks, hoop or ring tosses, darts, paddle boards, table tennis, golf ball putting, and croquet, and catching, batting or kicking a softball.

The Whitman children's game books (29) sold in variety stores are particularly well suited for amblyopia training. The books contain several interesting games of differing complexity, such as crossword puzzles, mazes, matching objects, completing a picture, coloring by number, detecting hidden figures, and joining dots of different sizes and separations. The games of Developmental Learning Materials (8), which include cutouts, tracing, jigsaws, and pegboard exercises, are also well suited for home amblyopia training.

Improvisations can be made, as circling letters in a newspaper or filling in the Os and Cs. Watching TV or motion pictures is helpful but tends to be too passive an exercise.

The *Visual Tracking Workbook* by Gaeke and Smith (2) is also applicable to amblyopia training. The book contains a series of paragraphs of meaningless grouped letters (make-believe words). The task is to read over the grouped letters and circle a letter the first time it appears in alphabetical sequence. Thus the first letter circled is the first *a* found, then the first *b* found, and so on until each letter in the alphabet is circled the first time it appears in the paragraph. The time required to complete the exercise is recorded after each paragraph has been completed. As the work progresses, the letters become smaller and more closely spaced. Special pens with disappearing ink may be used to make the books reusable.

The book *Monocular Vision Training* by Evans (30) is specifically designed for home training. It contains reading material in progressively smaller type and tracings of increasing complexity. The abridged English version of Sédan's *Re-Educative Treatment of Suppression Amblyopia* by Lyle et al. (14) is another such book. It contains reading exercises (proofreading and detecting errors), arithmetic and picture problems, and tracing exercises.

HYPNOTHERAPY

Performing visual training under hypnosis or under the influence of posthypnotic suggestion is an intriguing, though relatively unexplored, avenue of treating visual anomalies. By giving positive suggestions to one in a somnambulant state, it is conceivable that improvements may be elicited that otherwise would not be manifested.

The reports of Browning and Crasilneck (1957; with Quinn, 1958) and of Smith, Crasilneck and Browning (1961) on the use of post-hypnotic suggestion for the treatment of suppression amblyopia have indicated that hypnosis can produce improved acuity. Although the improvement obtained through posthypnotic suggestion tended to regress, significant increases in acuity on the subjects treated were obtained, especially at the near test distance.

It is a matter of conjecture as to how hypnosis effected this improvement. Was the acuity improvement due to a breakdown in synaptic inhibitions and a regaining of normal cortical reception and interpretation? Was it due to intensified cooperation and attention and a steadier fixation response? The basic question is this: Can hypnosis raise one's present maximum potential to a new and higher potential or does hypnosis serve to create a response equivalent to one's present maximum potential?

There is some reason to doubt that hypnosis can induce a neurological performance which is superior to the present neurological potential capability. A constant esotrope, for example, who does not have sensory fusion—that is, who cannot integrate and unify the impulses from the two eyes—will not be able to demonstrate this sensory skill through hypnosis. The neurological mechanism for sensory fusion is inoperable and remains inoperable.

There is no question, however, that hypnosis can be of great value in achieving maximum performance and in attaining cooperation, motivation, and even an eagerness to perform visual training exercises.

MEDICINAL THERAPY

Some limited attempts have been made in the application of drugs to break down synaptic inhibitions and thus increase the effectiveness of training to eliminate amblyopia. Bietti (1950, 1957; with Scorsonelli, 1955, 1956) found that producing a state of hyperoxia, either by having the patient breathe oxygen or by subconjunctivally injecting oxygen, reduced suppression influences. Bietti also obtained favorable results in using strychnine to increase visual sensitivity. Capobianco (1960), in applying the Bietti strychnine technique, reported it to be most effective when the visual reduction was mild, fixation central, or when the amblyopia was associated with anisometropia and not strabismus.

Amobarbital, a sedative or hypnotic drug used in psychiatry in narcoanalysis to remove psychic suppression, was used by Tsutsui (1966) to combat suppression in amblyopia and enhance the effectiveness of pleoptics. The visual acuity improvement attained was superior to that with pleoptics alone, although the drug did not affect fixation behavior.

The beneficial effect of amobarbital is attributed to its removal of suppression and the resulting increase in conductivity of impulses along the visual pathway. Tsutsui suggests that this drug acts either in the lateral geniculate body or in the reticular system. The injection of the drug produced an immediate, though temporary, increase in acuity in functional amblyopia, but not in organic amblyopia. It thus may be of value in the differential diagnosis of these two types of amblyopia.

Patterns of Improvement

Improvement manifestations resulting from occlusion and visual training vary greatly from individual to individual. As a rule, acuity and fixation improve rapidly during the first weeks of treatment and then gradually slow before reaching a plateau (Byron, 1960; Wild, 1961). On occasion, however, improvement occurs at a relatively slow and even pace (von Noorden, 1964), this being particularly true of older children or adults.

There is a tendency for single-letter acuity to improve faster than line acuity (von Noorden, 1964); in some instances, single-letter acuity may improve to near normal while line acuity remains essentially unchanged (Matteuci, 1960). Also, near-point acuity may improve faster than far-point acuity (Mayweg and Massie, 1958).

Acuity increases do not necessarily occur simultaneously with improvement in fixation and spatial localization. Although steady, pursuit, and saccadic fixations tend to become steadier and smoother (Mackensen, 1957; von Noorden, 1964), the basic fixation pattern may remain unchanged even though a significant acuity improvement is attained (Wheeler, 1956; Priestley, 1960; von Noorden, 1964). This may be attributed to steadier fixation and to a breakdown of synaptic inhibitions with resulting improved cortical reception and interpretation of impulses derived from the same retinal area. Spatial localization and hand-eye coordination may also continue to be anomalous despite acuity improvement (Matteucci, 1960).

Conversely, the fixation pattern may improve while acuity increase lags (Byron, 1960; Priestley, 1960; von Noorden, 1964). This may be attributed to the emphasis on eccentric fixation in the Bangerter and Cüppers methods. As a result, these pleoptic techniques are more successful in restoring centric fixation than in restoring acuity (Wild, 1961; von Noorden, 1964).

The achievement of 20/20 acuity, in fact, is not a common or typical occurrence (Wheeler, 1956; Wild, 1961; von Noorden, 1964). Although the majority do show significant acuity improvement, few reach the 20/20 level. No doubt the primary factor involved for the lack of success in establishing 20/20 acuity relates to the age of onset and the duration of the condition leading to amblyopia ex anopsia. If training or corrective procedures could be initiated at the very early age levels (4 or younger), the establishment of 20/20 acuity would be the rule rather than the exception. The younger in life the condition starts and the longer it is permitted to exist untreated, the more resistant will it be to treatment, and the poorer the prognosis for complete recovery of function.

The level of acuity achieved at the conclusion of the training period is frequently found to regress thereafter. The reported incidence of acuity regression varies between one fourth and one half (Hammer, 1956; Gale, 1957; Wild, 1961; von Noorden, 1964).

Although that is discouraging, it should not be unexpected. Treatment to eliminate amblyopia is generally the initial step in a training program whose ultimate objective is the establishment of normal binocular vision, free from fixation anomalies and central suppression. Should fixation anomalies and/or suppression persist, the cause of the amblyopia remains present and operative and a reduction of acuity should be anticipated.

Regressions in strabismic amblyopia are especially common if training fails to eliminate the binocular anomalies accompanying strabismus. So there is some question about the advisability of instituting acuity training for strabismic amblyopia if the prognosis for the eventual cure of the strabismus is poor: strabismus cannot be eliminated and acuity improvement regresses when treatment is discontinued.

The point is valid and must be faced realistically when accepting patients for training. If one holds to this view, amblyopia training is recommended only for those patients who are likely to retain the acuity improvement. Hence, in addition to the factors of cooperation, motivation and age, strabismics selected for acuity training should offer a reasonably good prognosis for the restoration of normal binocular vision.

In contrast to that is the belief that acuity training is desirable and should be given even if it is likely that acuity will regress after cessation of training. The logic for this position is that the amblyopic eye may be considered a spare or reserve eye which someday may be used in the event of disease or trauma to the currently fixating eye. The visual acuity improvement achieved through training, even though it regresses, is potentially recoverable should vision become dependent upon the amblyopic eye. Some even recommend that periodic training be given to such patients to maintain acuity in the amblyopic eye at the highest possible level (Priestley, Byron and Weseley, 1959).

Another consideration relates to the accuracy with which one can predict whether or not binocular vision can be established. Effectively administered training to eliminate amblyopia, fixation anomalies and suppression may result in binocular vision, though the prognosis is believed poor.

Prognosticating the results of visual training is, in effect, an evaluation of chances of success in terms of percentage cures for that type of visual problem. Although the percentage of success may be low, the only sure way to determine if training will be productive is to make the attempt.

Suppliers of Optical
Instruments and Materials

1. American Optical Corporation, 14 Mechanic St., Southbridge, Massachusetts 01550.
2. Ann Arbor Publishers, 611 Church Street, Ann Arbor, Michigan 48104.
3. Armco Mercantile Company, 7 West Madison Street, Chicago, Illinois 60602.
4. Bausch & Lomb, Inc., 635 St. Paul Street, Rochester, New York 14602.
5. Bernell Corporation, 316 South Eddy Street, South Bend, Indiana 46617.
6. Clement Clarke, Ltd., Instrument Division, Wigmore Street, London W. 1, England.
7. Cortland Optical Company, Ogdensburg, New York.
8. Developmental Learning Materials, 3505 North Ashland Avenue, Chicago, Illinois 60657.
9. Good-Lite Company, 7426 Madison Street, Forest Park, Illinois 60130.
10. House of Vision, Inc., 137 North Wabash Avenue, Chicago, Illinois 60602.
11. Keeler Optical Products, Inc., 5536 Baltimore Avenue, Philadelphia, Pennsylvania 19143.
12. Kelley & Hueber, Inc., 5235 Whitby Avenue, Philadelphia, Pennsylvania 19143.
13. Keystone View Company, Hamilton and Crandall Streets, Meadville, Pennsylvania 16335.
14. E. and S. Livingstone, Ltd., Edinburgh and London.
15. Long Island Orthoptic Instrument Company, 3 Collingwood Drive, Huntington Station, New York 11747.
16. Medical Charts and Specialties Company (J. L. Krause), Box 211, Glenview, Illinois.
17. Metropolitan Optical Supply, 42 Barton Avenue, Westmount, Montreal 6, Quebec, Canada.
18. National Foundation for Educational Research, 79 Wimpole Street, London W 1, England.
19. Neefe Optical Company, Big Springs, Texas.

20. Neitz Instruments Co., Ltd., Taneker Bldg. No. 23, Honshiocho Shinjuku-ku, Tokyo, Japan.
21. Oculus Products, Dutenhofen, Federal Republic of Germany.
22. Alfred P. Poll, Inc., 40 W. 55th Street, New York, New York 10019.
23. Ophthalmix, Inc., La Grange, Illinois.
24. Stercks Martin, Ltd., 56 New Cavendish Street, London, WIM 7LE, England.
25. AB Stille-Werner, Stockholm, Sweden.
26. University of California Optometry Alumni Association, Special Projects Committee, Berkeley, California 94720.
27. Western Optical Company, 1200 Mercer Street, Seattle, Washington 98109
28. Whitman Publishing Company, 1220 Mound Avenue, Racine, Wisconsin 53404.
29. Williams & Wilkins Company, 428 East Preston Street, Baltimore, Maryland 21202.

Bibliography

Abraham, S. V., The nature of heterophorias, *American Journal of Orth.*, 34 (7):1007–1016, 1951.

———, Accommodation in the amblyopic eye, *American Journal of Ophthalmology*, 52(2):197–199, 1961.

———, Bilateral ametropic amblyopia, *Journal of Pediatric Ophthalmology*, 1(1):57–61, 1964.

———, *Nonparalytic Strabismus, Amblyopia and Heterophoria.* Pan-American Publishing Co., 1966.

Adler, Francis H., *Gifford's Textbook of Ophthalmology*, 6th ed. Philadelphia, W. B. Saunders Co., 1957.

———, *Physiology of the Eye: Clinical Application*, St. Louis, Mo., C. V. Mosby Co., 3rd ed., 1959; 4th ed., 1965.

———, Foveal fixation, *American Journal of Ophthalmology*, 56(3, pt. I):483–484, 1963.

——— and M. Fliegelman, Influence of fixation on the visual acuity, *Archives of Ophthalmology*, 12(4):475–483, 1934.

——— and G. Meyer, Mechanism of the fovea, *Transactions of the American Ophthalmological Society*, 33:266, 1935.

Agarwal, L. P., P. Prakash, S. R. K. Malik, and M. Mohan, Pleoptics in amblyopia with eccentric fixation, *Oriental Archives of Ophthalmology*, 1:39–44, 1963.

Agatston, H., Ocular malingering, *Archives of Ophthalmology*, 31(3):223–231, 1944.

D'Agostino, A., and M. D'Esposito, Examination of the monocular central visual field and the visual acuity with a telescopic lens for prognosis in amblyopia, *Archivio di Ottalmologia*, 66:307–321, July–Aug., 1962.

Allen, H. F., A new picture series for preschool vision testing, *American Journal of Ophthalmology*, 44(1):38–41, 1957.

Allen, Merrill J., The Bartley phenomenon and visual rehabilitation—a home training technique, *Optometric Weekly*, 57(30):21–22, 1966.

Alpern, M., D. B. Flitman, and R. H. Joseph, Centrally fixed flicker thresholds in amblyopia, *American Journal of Ophthalmology*, 49(5, pt. II): 1194–1202, 1960.

———, R. R. Petrauskas, G. S. Sandall, and R. J. Vorenkamp, Recent experiments on the physiology of strabismus amblyopia, *American Orthoptic Journal,* 17:62–72, 1967.

Ambrose, D. A., Conditioned tonotic treatment and macular generation, *Optometric Weekly,* 53(35):1712–1714, 1962.

Ammann, E., Einige Beobachtunger bei den Funktionsprüfungen in der Sprechstunde: "zentrales" Sehen-Sehen der Glaukomatösen-Sehen der Amblyopen, *Klinische Monatsblätter für Augenheilkunde,* 66:564–573, 1921.

Arruga, A., Effect of occlusion of the amblyopic eye on amblyopia and eccentric fixation, *Transactions of the Ophthalmological Society of the United Kingdom,* 82:45–61, 1962.

――――, The role of prophylactic occlusion in amblyopia, *Archivos de la Sociedad oftalmológica hispano-americana,* 24:105–110, 1964.

―――― and R. Downey, Simple modification of synoptophore; useful in pleoorthoptic treatment, *American Journal of Ophthalmology,* 50(1): 156–158, 1960.

Aubert, H., and R. Förster, Beiträge zur Kenntniss des indirekte Sehens (I) Untersuchungen über den Raumsinn der Retina, *Albrecht von Graefe's Archiv für Ophthalmologie,* 3:1–37, 1857.

Aulhorn, E., Relations between light sense and visual acuity, *Albrecht von Graefe's Archiv für Ophthalmologie,* 167:4–74, 1964.

Backman, H. A., Pleoptics, *Optica International,* 3(1):6–22, 1966.

Baldwin, W. R., Pleoptics: historical developments and review of the literature, *American Journal of Optometry and Archives of American Academy of Optometry,* 39(3):149–162, 1962.

van Balen, A. T. M., and H. E. Henkes, Attention and amblyopia, an electro-encephalographic approach to an ophthalmological problem, *British Journal of Ophthalmology,* 46(1):12–20, 1962.

Bangerter, A., *Amblyopiebehandlung.* Basel, Switzerland, S. Karger, 1953; 2nd ed., 1955.

――――, Über Pleoptik, *Wiener Klinische Wochenschrift,* 65:966, 1953.

――――, Kapitel aus der Pleoptik un Orthoptik, *Ophthalmologica,* 129(4–5): 237–240, 1955.

――――, Die Okklusion in der Pleoptik und Orthoptik, *Klinische Monatsblätter für Augenheilkunde,* 136(3):305–331, 1960.

――――, Notre devoir envers les enfants amblyopes, *Bulletins et Memoires de la Société française d'Ophtalmologie,* 62(5):332–340, 1962.

Bárány, E. H., and U. Halldén, The influence of some central nervous depressants on the reciprocal inhibition between the two retinae as manifested in retinal rivalry, *Acta Physiologica Scandinavica,* 14:296–316, 1947.

―――― and ――――, Phasic inhibition of the light reflex of the pupil during retinal rivalry, *Journal of Neurophysiology,* 11:25–30, 1948.

Barnard, W., Treatment of amblyopia by inverse occlusion and pleoptics, *British Orthoptic Journal,* 19:19–30, 1962.

Barraquer, J. I., E. Ariza, and S. Reinoso, Our experience in treatment of the amblyopia by the method of after-images, *Archivos de la Sociedad Americana de Oftalmologia y Optometria,* 1(1):58–73, 1958.

Bartley, S. Howard, *Principles of Perception,* 2nd ed. New York, Harper and Row, Publishers, 1969.

Beale, J. P., Current concepts and treatment of amblyopia, *American Orthoptic Journal,* 11:101–108, 1961.

Belostotsky, E., and F. Friedman, The treatment of amblyopia in false light fixation, *Vestnik Oftalmologii,* 6:18–23, 1957.

Bessière, Chabot (Mme.), Dutertre (and) Mirande, Utilisations sémiologiques de l'adaptometrie et de l'électroretinographie, *Bulletin des Sociétés d'Ophtalmologie de France,* 10:706–714, 1957.

———, ———, ——— (and) ———, Lesions muculaires différenciées par l'électroretinographie et l'adaptometrie, *Bulletin des Sociétés d'Ophtalmologie de France,* 10:715–718, 1957.

Bielschowsky, A., Über monoculäre Diplopie ohne physikalische Grundlage nebst Bemerkungen über das Sehen schielender, *Albrecht von Graefe's Archiv für Ophthalmologie,* 46:143–183, 1898.

Bietti, G. B., L'action de l'oxygène sur les fonctions rétiniennes: son emploi en clinique, *Bulletins et Mémoires de la Société française d'Ophtalmologie,* 63:195–210, 1950.

———, Sur la possibilité d'un traitement médicamenteux des phénomènes suppressifs en vision binoculaire dans le strabisme, *Mod. Probl. Ophthal.,* 1:391–404, 1957.

——— and B. Bagolini, Present status and comments on pleoptics and orthoptics, *Journal of Pediatric Ophthalmology,* 2(1):7–20, 1965.

——— and M. Scorsonelli, Azione del'O₂ sui fenomeni di suppressione in visione binoculare degli strabici, *Revista de Medicina Aeronautica,* 18(1):23–67, 1955.

——— and ———, Indagini sulla possibilità di un trattamento medicamentosa dei fenomeni di soppressione in visione binoculare degli strabici, *Atti XII Cong. Soc. oftal. ital.,* 15:88–95, 1955, published 1956.

Binder, H. F., Management of recurrent amblyopia, *American Orthoptic Journal,* 9:111–113, 1959.

———, D. Engel, M. L. Ede, and L. Loon, The red filter treatment of eccentric fixation, *American Orthoptic Journal,* 13:64–69, 1963.

Bishop, J. W., Treatment of amblyopia secondary to anisometropia, *British Orthoptic Journal,* 14:68–74, 1957.

Böhme, G., Zur Kenntnis der exzentrischen Fixation im Hinblick auf die Behandlung der Amblyopie, *Klinische Monatsblätter für Augenheilkunde,* 126(6):694–719, 1955.

———. Über die motorische Komponente der exzentrischen Fixation und ihre operative Korrektur, *Klinische Monatsblätter für Augenheilkunde,* 130(5):628–637, 1957.

Borish, I. M., *Clinical Refraction,* 2nd ed. Chicago, Professional Press, Inc., 1954.

Bourquin, A., L'incidence des maladies sur les yeux amblyopes, *Ophthalmologica*, 125(6):405–409, 1953.

Brattgård, S.-O., The importance of adequate stimulation for the chemical composition of retinal ganglion cells during early postnatal development, *Acta Radiologica*, (Stockholm), Suppl. 96:1–80, 1952.

Brinker, W. R., and S. L. Katz, A new and practical treatment of eccentric fixation, *American Journal of Ophthalmology*, 55(5):1033–1035, 1963.

Brock, Frederick W., Monocular amblyopia, *Optometric Weekly*, 34(42): 1209–1214, 1943.

———, Visual training, *Optometric Weekly*, 41(46):1702, 1715–1719, 1950; 42(19):747–756, 1951; 42(34):1331–1349, 1951; 42(39): 1517–1522, 1951; 43(41):1641–1645, 1952; 43(42):1683–1687, 1952.

———, *Visual training*, Pt. 2. Chicago, Professional Press, Inc., 1953.

———, Factors in the management of amblyopic and strabismic patients, *Optometric Weekly*, 53(33):1617–1621, 1962.

———, Investigation of the fovea centralis in amblyopia, *American Journal of Ophthalmology*, 54(5):821–827, 1962.

———, A chronicle of orthoptic history covering 25 years of practice, *Optometric Weekly*, 57(7):23–27, 1966.

———, The care of the amblyopic child—an overview, *American Journal of Optometry and Archives of American Academy of Optometry*, 44(1):42–55, 1967.

——— and I. Givner, Fixation anomalies in amblyopia, *Archives of Ophthalmology*, 47(6):775–786, 1952.

——— and J. Schechter, Minute monocular central scotoma, *Optometric Weekly*, 32(52):1465–1466, 1942.

Brockbank, G., and R. Downey, Measurement of eccentric fixation by the Bjerrum screen, *British Journal of Ophthalmology*, 43(8):461–470, 1959.

Brown, F. G., Pleoptics, *British Journal of Physiological Optics*, 22(2):91–113, 1965.

Browning, C. W., and H. B. Crasilneck, The experimental use of hypnosis in suppression amblyopia, *American Journal of Ophthalmology*, 44(4 Pt. 1):468–476, 1957.

———, L. H. Quinn, and H. B. Crasilneck, The use of hypnosis in suppression amblyopia of children, *American Journal of Ophthalmology*, 46(1 Pt. 1):53–67, 1958.

Bryngdahl, O., Effect of retinal image motion on visual acuity, *Optica Acta*, 8(1):1–16, 1961.

deBuffon, G. L., Sur le cause du strabisme ou des yeux louches, *Mémoires de l'Academie des Sciences*, Paris, 1743 (cited by William S. Smith, Clinical Orthoptic Procedure, 2nd ed., 1954, p. 277).

Bullock, K., Treatment of eccentric fixation by the red filter method, *British Opthoptic Journal*, 21:83–84, 1964.

Burian, H. M., Adaptive mechanisms, *Transactions of the American Academy of Ophthalmology and Otolaryngology,* 57(2):131–144, 1953.

———, Thoughts on the nature of amblyopia ex anopsia, *American Orthoptic Journal,* 6:5–12, 1956.

———, Treatment of amblyopia ex anopsia with eccentric fixation, *Journal of the Iowa State Medical Society,* August:449–455, 1956.

———, Occlusion amblyopia, *American Journal of Ophthalmology,* 62(5): 853–856, 1966.

———, A. L. Benton, and R. C. Lipsius, Visual cognitive functions in patients with strabismic amblyopia, *Archives of Ophthalmology,* 68(6):785–791, 1962.

——— and R. M. Cortimiglia, Visual acuity and fixation pattern in patients with strabismic amblyopia, *American Orthoptic Journal,* 12:169–174, 1962.

——— and T. Lawwill, Electroretinographic studies in strabismic amblyopia, *American Journal of Ophthalmology,* 61(3):422–430, 1966.

——— and C. W. Watson, Cerebral electric response to intermittent photic stimulation in amblyopia ex anopsia: a preliminary report, *Archives of Ophthalmology,* 48(8):137–143, 1952.

Byram, G. M., The physical and photochemical basis of visual resolving power: II, visual acuity and the photochemistry of the retina, *Journal of the Optical Society of America,* 34(12):718–738, 1944.

Byron, H. M., Results of pleoptics in the management of amblyopia with eccentric fixation, *Archives of Ophthalmology,* 63(4):675–681, 1960.

Callahan, W. P., Investigation of amblyopia, *Transactions of the Canadian Ophthalmological Society,* 24:186–195, 1961.

Caloroso, E., and M. C. Flom, Visual acuity in amblyopia: influence of retinal locus and luminance. Paper read before the annual meeting of the American Academy of Optometry, Chicago, Dec. 9, 1967.

——— and ———, Influence of luminance on visual acuity in amblyopia, *American Journal of Optometry and Archives of American Academy of Optometry,* 46(3):189–195, 1969.

Campbell, F. W., and A. H. Gregory, The spatial resolving power of the human retina with oblique incidence (letter to the Editor), *Journal of the Optical Society of America,* 50(8):831, 1960.

Campos, E., Optotypes for small children, *Revista brasileira de Oftalmología,* 22:265–269, 1963.

Cantrell, G. L., Near vision testing in young children, *British Orthoptic Journal,* 21:68–72, 1964.

Capobianco, N. M., Pleoptic treatment of amblyopes with central and eccentric fixation, *American Orthoptic Journal,* 10:33–53, 1960.

Carifa, R. P., and F. W. Hebbard, Involuntary eye movements occurring during fixation: effects of changes in target contrast, *American Journal of Optometry and Archives of American Academy of Optometry,* 44(2):73–90, 1967.

Carroll, F. D., The etiology and treatment of tobacco-alcohol amblyopia,

American Journal of Ophthalmology, Part I, 27(7):713–725; Part II, 27(7):847–863, 1944.

Catford, G. V., A comparison between distance and near vision, *British Journal of Ophthalmology*, 40:633–635, 1956.

Chambers, R., and A. A. Cinotti, Functional disorders of central vision, *American Journal of Ophthalmology*, 59(6):1091–1095, 1965.

Chavasse, F. Bernard, *Worth's Squint*, 7th ed. Philadelphia, Pa., Blakiston's Son and Co., Inc., 1939.

Chinaglia, V., and B. Andreani, Consideragioni sui risultati dell'occlusione nell'ambliopia strabica, *Annali di Ottalmologia e Clinica Oculistica*, 81(12):563–574, 1955.

Cholst, M. R., I. J. Cohen, and M. A. Losty, Evaluation of amblyopia problem in the child, *New York State Journal of Medicine*, 62(12): 3927–3930, 1962.

Chow, K. L., Failure to demonstrate changes in the visual system of monkeys kept in darkness or in colored lights, *Journal of Comparative Neurology*, 102(6):597–606, 1955.

———, A. H. Riesen, and F. W. Newell, Degeneration of retinal ganglion cells in infant chimpanzees reared in darkness, *Journal of Comparative Neurology*, 107:27–42, 1957.

Cibis, L., and C. Windsor, Clinical results with passive amblyopia treatment, *American Orthoptic Journal*, 17:56–61, 1967.

Clark, W. E. LeGros, The laminar organization and cell content of the lateral geniculate body in the monkey, *Journal of Anatomy*, 75(Pt. 4):419–433, 1941.

Clerici, A., and L. Legorini, Artificial scotoma as therapy in amblyopia with abnormal fixation, *Archivio di Ottalmologia*, 59:285–316, 1955.

Cole, R. B. W., The problem of unilateral amblyopia, *British Medical Journal*, 1(1):202–206, 1959.

Costenbader, F. D., D. G. Albert, and R. L. Hiatt, Some thoughts about strabismus, in *The Year Book of Ophthalmology, 1963–1964 Series*, edited by W. F. Hughes, Chicago, Year Book Medical Publishers, Inc., 1964.

———, D. Bair, and A. McPhail, Vision in strabismus; a preliminary report, *Archives of Ophthalmology*, 40(10):438–453, 1948.

Cowan, L. J., M. M. Bennet, and D. K. Ogg, Diagnostic and therapeutic uses of filters in orthoptics and pleoptics, *American Orthoptic Journal*, 16:24–29, 1966.

Cowle, J. B., J. H. Kunst, and A. M. Philpotts, Trial with red filter in the treatment of eccentric fixation, *British Journal of Ophthalmology*, 51(3):165–168, 1967.

Crane, H. D., Automatic focus by the human eye, *Optometric Weekly*, 57(33):36–41, 1966.

Cristini, G., The physiopathological cerebral basis of inhibition and amblyopia, of anomalous correspondence and eccentric fixation in concomitant squint, *Ophthalmologica*, 143(1):15–19, 1962.

Cunningham, F., Preschool vision screening, *American Journal of Public Health*, 49:762–765, 1959.

Cüppers, C., Die Amblyopiebehandlung mit der Nachbildmethode, *Wissenschaftliche Zeitschrift der Universität Jena, Mathematisch-natuurwissenschaftliche Reihe*, 5:21, 1956.

——, Moderne Schielbehandlung, *Klinische Monatsblätter für Augenheilkunde*, 129(5):579–604, 1956.

——, *Orthoptic and Pleoptic Problems in Germany*, Lecture before the North of England Ophthalmological Society, June 12 and 13, 1958. Printed by Wm. Foster and Sons, Ltd.

——, Grenzen und Möglichkeiten der pleoptischen Therapie, *in Schiel-Pleoptik-Orthoptik-Operation*. Stuttgart, Ferdinand Enke Verlag, 1961.

——, Problèmes de fixation, *Bulletins et Mémoires de la Société française d'Ophtalmologie*, 62(9):309–316, 1962.

——, Therapie der Amblyopie und des concomitiererden Schielens an der Giessner Augenklinik, *Giessener Medizinische*, Nov.:2–6, 1964.

Daily, R. K., and L. Daily, The modern techniques in the treatment of amblyopia, *American Orthoptic Journal*, 9:36–42, 1959.

Davson, Hugh, *The Eye*, Vol. 2: *The Visual Process*. New York, Academic Press, Inc., 1962.

Dayton, G. O., Jr., G. Jensen, and M. H. Jones, Visual Acuity of infants measured by means of optokinetic nystagmus and oculogram, *Investigative Ophthalmology*, 1(3):414, 1962.

——, M. H. Jones, P. Aiu, R. A. Rawson, B. Steele, and M. Rose, Developmental study of coordinated eye movements in the human infant. I. Visual acuity in the newborn: A study based on induced optokinetic nystagmus recorded by electro-oculography, *Archives of Ophthalmology*, 71(6):865–870, 1964.

——, ——, B. Steele, and M. Rose, Developmental study of coordinated eye movements in the human infant. II. An electro-oculographic study of the fixation reflex in the newborn, *Archives of Ophthalmology*, 71(6):871–875, 1964.

DeRuchie, C., Suppression amblyopia, *Optometric Weekly*, 98(47):2205–2210, 1957.

Dolénk, A., A. Křístek, J. Němec, and S. Komenda, Über Veränderungen der Pupillenreaktion nach erfolgreicher Amblyopiebehandlung, *Klinische Monatsblätter für Augenheilkunde*, 141(9):353–357, 1962.

Dossi, F., and L. Luizzi, Electroretinography in strabismic amblyopia, *Rassegna italiana d'Ottalmologia*, 31:119–127, 1962.

Douthwaite, C. M., Orthoptics in Lyons, *British Orthoptic Journal*, 14:56–60, 1957.

—— and B. Lee, An investigation of pleoptics at the High Holborn Branch of the Moorfields Eye Hospital, *British Orthoptic Journal*, 15:27–35, 1958.

Downey, R., New ideas gleaned in foreign clinics for the treatment of amblyopia, especially that due to eccentric fixation, *British Orthoptic Journal*, 14:47–52, 1957.

———, Amblyopia, *British Orthoptic Journal*, 15:36–54, 1958.

Downing, A. H., Ocular defects in sixty thousand selectees, *Archives of Ophthalmology*, 33(2):137–143, 1945.

Dreyfus, P. M., Blood transketolase levels in tobacco-alcohol amblyopia, *Archives of Ophthalmology*, 74(5):617–620, 1965.

Duke-Elder, Stewart, *Textbook of Ophthalmology*. St. Louis, Mo., C. V. Mosby Co., Vol. 3, 1941; Vol. 4, 1949.

———, *System of Ophthalmology*, Vol. III, Pt. 2, *Congenital Deformities*. St. Louis, Mo., C. V. Mosby Co., 1963.

Dyer, D., and E. O. Bierman, Cortical potential changes in amblyopia ex anopsia, *American Journal of Ophthalmology*, 33(7):1095–1098, 1950.

——— and ———, Cortical potential changes in suppression amblyopia, *American Journal of Ophthalmology*, 35(1):66–68, 1952.

Ehrich, W., The separating difficulties of the amblyopic eye: their diagnosis and therapeutic training by means of a new device, *Klinische Monatsblätter für Augenheilkunde*, 127:221–224, 1955.

———, Der Einfluss der Schieloperation auf den Fixationsort des Amblyopen Auges, *Klinische Monatsblätter für Augenheilkunde*, 133(6):846–848, 1958.

———, Muskelsensibilität und Fixation, *Albrecht von Graefe's Archiv für Ophthalmologie*, 161(11):185–191, 1959.

Enoch, J. M., Amblyopia and the Stiles-Crawford effect, *American Journal of Optometry and Archives of American Academy of Optometry*, 34(6):298–309, 1957.

———, Further studies on the relationship between amblyopia and the Stiles-Crawford effect, *American Journal of Optometry and Archives of American Academy of Optometry*, 36(3):111–128, 1959.

———, Receptor amblyopia, *American Journal of Ophthalmology*, 48(3 Pt. II): 262–274, 1959.

Enos, M. V., Suppression versus amblyopia, *American Journal of Ophthalmology*, 27(11):1266–1271, 1944.

Evans, M. S., *Monocular Vision Training*. Baltimore, Williams & Wilkins Company, 1946.

Fantz, R. L., A method of studying depth perception in infants under six months of age, *Psych. Rec.*, 11:27–32, 1961.

———, The origin of form perception, *Scientific American*, 204(5):66–72, 1961.

———, Pattern vision in newborn infants, *Science*, 140:296–297, 1963.

——— and J. M. Ordy, A visual acuity test for infants under six months of age, *Psych. Rec.*, 9:159–164, 1959.

———, ——— and M. S. Udelf, Maturation of pattern vision in infants during the first six months, *Journal of Comparative and Physiological Psychology*, 55(6):907–917, 1962.

Feinberg, I., Critical flicker frequency in amblyopia ex anopsia, *American Journal of Ophthalmology*, 42(3):473–481, 1956.

Feinberg, R., A study of some aspects of peripheral visual acuity, *American Journal of Optometry and Archives of American Academy of Optometry*, 26(2):49–56, 1949.

Feldman, J. B., Further studies in amblyopia, *American Journal of Ophthalmology*, 32(10):1394–1398, 1949.

―――― and A. F. Taylor, Obstacle to squint training—amblyopia, *Archives of Ophthalmology*, 27(5):851–868, 1942.

Fender, D., Control mechanisms of the eye, *Scientific American*, 211(7):24–33, 1964.

Fitton, M. H., Pleoptics in the U. S. A., *British Orthoptic Journal*, 19:35–38, 1962.

Flax, N., Pleoptics and functional optometry, *Optical Journal and Review of Optometry*, XCVIII(17):27–30, 1961.

Flom, M. C., The University of California strabismus and orthoptics study; a preliminary report. (Unpublished paper cited with personal permission of the author.)

――――, A minimum strabismus examination, *Journal of the American Optometric Association*, 27(5):642–649, 1956.

――――, New concepts in visual acuity, *Optometric Weekly*, 57(28):63–68, 1966.

――――, G. G. Heath, and E. Takaháshi, Contour interaction and visual resolution: contralateral effects, *Science*, 142(3594):979–980, 1963.

―――― and K. E. Kerr, Amblyopia: a hidden threat? *Journal of the American Optometric Association*, 36(10):906–912, 1965.

―――― and R. W. Neumaier, Prevalence of amblyopia, *American Journal of Optometry and Archives of American Academy of Optometry*, 43(11): 732–751, 1966.

―――― and F. W. Weymouth, Centricity of Maxwell's spot in strabismus and amblyopia, *Archives of Ophthalmology*, 66(2):260–268, 1961.

――――, ――――, and D. Kahneman, Visual resolution and contour interaction, *Journal of the Optical Society of America*, 53(9):1026–1032, 1963.

Flynn, J. T., Spatial summation in amblyopia, *Archives of Ophthalmology*, 78(4):470–474, 1967.

――――, Dark adaptation in amblyopia, *Archives of Ophthalmology*, 79(6): 697–704, 1968.

Fonda, G. E., Method of testing visual acuity in the amblyopic eye, *American Orthoptic Journal*, 8:149–150, 1958.

Foster, J., Contribution to discussion on pleoptics, *British Orthoptic Journal*, 14:53–55, 1957.

Fowler, F., The treatment of amblyopia, *American Orthoptic Journal*, 6:19–28, 1956.

François, J., and M. James, Comparative study on amblyopic treatment, *American Orthoptic Journal*, 5:61–64, 1955.

—————— and G. Verriest, The visual functions in strabismic amblyopia, *Journal of Pediatric Ophthalmology,* 2(4):59–64, 1965.

Freedman, N. L., Bilateral differences in the human occipital electroencephalogram with unilateral photic driving, *Science,* 142(11):598–599, 1963.

Frezzotti, R., and E. Nucci, Osservazioni elettroretinografiche nell'ambliopia, *Giornale italiano di Oftalmologia,* 11:199–203, 1958.

Friensen, H., and W. A. Mann, Follow-up study of hysterical amblyopia, *American Journal of Ophthalmology,* 62(6):1106–1115, 1966.

Gale, H., Pleoptics, *British Orthoptic Journal,* 14:43–46, 1957.

Gibson, H. W., *Textbook of Orthoptics.* London, Hatton Press, Ltd., 1955.

Giles, G. H., *The Practice of Orthoptics.* London, Hammond, Hammond & Co., Ltd., 1945.

Girard, L. J., M. C. Fletcher, E. Tomlinson, and B. Smith, Results of pleoptic treatment of suppression amblyopia, *American Orthoptic Journal,* 12:12–31, 1962.

Glover, L. P., and W. R. Brewer, An ophthalmologic review of more than twenty thousand men at the Altoona Induction Center, *American Journal of Ophthalmology,* 27(4):346–348, 1944.

Goldschmidt, M., A new test for function of the macula lutea, *Archives of Ophthalmology,* 44(1):129–135, 1950.

Goldstein, H. J., J. A. Katko, and R. W. Zehner, Predicting the success of training amblyopes, *American Journal of Optometry and Archives of American Academy of Optometry,* 32(1):3–9, 1955.

Goodman, L., Effect of total absence of function on the optic system of rabbits, *American Journal of Physiology,* 100:46–63, 1932.

Gording, E. J., A report on Haidinger brushes, *American Journal of Optometry and Archives of American Academy of Optometry,* 27(12):604–610, 1950.

Gorman, J. J., D. G. Cogan, and S. S. Gellis, An apparatus for grading the visual acuity of infants on the basis of optokinetic nystagmus, *Pediatrics,* 19(6):1088–1092, 1957.

Görtz, H., The corrective treatment of amblyopia with eccentric fixation, *American Journal of Ophthalmology,* 49(6):1315–1321, 1960.

Graham, Clarence H. (ed.), *Vision and Visual Perception.* New York, John Wiley & Sons, Inc., 1965.

Green, D. G., Visual resolution when light enters the eye through different parts of the pupil, *Journal of Physiology,* 190(3):583–593, 1967.

Grosvenor, T., The effects of duration and background luminance upon the brightness discrimination of an amblyope, *American Journal of Optometry and Archives of American Academy of Optometry,* 34(12):639–663, 1957.

Guzzinati, G. C., Anisometropia e visione binoculare, *Bollettino d' Oculistica,* 36(4):219–234, 1957.

Halldén, U., An explanation of Haidinger's brushes, *Archives of Ophthalmology,* 57(3):393–399, 1957.

Hammer, J., Results of squint treatment—final results? *Klinische Monatsblätter für Augenheilkunde*, 128(2):195–199, 1956.

Harada, H., and S. Hayashi, Differential diagnosis of amblyopia, *Japanese Journal of Ophthalmology*, 2(4):268–273, 1958.

Hardesty, H. H., Occlusion amblyopia, *Archives of Ophthalmology*, 62(2): 314–316, 1959.

Harms, H., Ort und Wesen der Bildemmung bei Schielenden, *Albrecht von Graefe's Archiv für Ophthalmologie*, 138:149–210, 1938.

Harrington, David O., *The Visual Fields*. St. Louis, Mo., C. V. Mosby Co., 1956.

———, Amblyopia due to tobacco, alcohol, and nutritional deficiency, *American Journal of Ophthalmology*, 53(6):967–972, 1962.

Hauser, P. J., Studies on the fixation patterns in amblyopia ex anopsia, *American Journal of Ophthalmology*, 41(6):1073–1074, 1956.

——— and H. M. Burian, Fixation patterns in strabismic amblyopia, *Archives of Ophthalmology*, 57(2):254–258, 1957.

Havener, W. H., and W. R. Harris, The management of suppression amblyopia, *American Orthoptic Journal*, 10:5–14, 1961.

Haynes, H., B. L. White, and R. Held, Visual accommodation in human infants, *Science*, 148(3669):528–530, 1965.

Haynes, P. R., The physiological basis for the prescribing of occluders in the treatment of amblyopia, *American Journal of Optometry and Archives of American Academy of Optometry*, 34(8):417–421, 1956.

Heaton, J. M., Chronic cyanide poisoning and optic neuritis, *Transactions of the Ophthalmological Society of the United Kingdom*, 82:263, 1962.

Hebbard, F. W., Eye Movements During Fixation and Fusion. Unpublished Ph.D. thesis, Berkeley, University of California, 1957.

———, A new method of recording small eye movements using corneal reflections, *American Journal of Optometry and Archives of American Academy of Optometry*, 41(4):241–247, 1964.

Hecht, S., and E. U. Mintz, The visibility of single lines at various illuminations and the retinal basis of visual resolution, *Journal of General Physiology*, 22:593–612, 1939.

Helveston, E. M., The incidence of amblyopia ex anopsia in young adult males in Minnesota in 1962–63, *American Journal of Ophthalmology*, 60(1):75–77, 1965.

———, Relationship between degree of anisometropia and depth of amblyopia, *American Journal of Ophthalmology*, 62(4):757–759, 1966.

Henao, H., Amblyopic treatment by means of pleoptics, *Archives de la Sociedad Americana de Oftalmologia y Optometria*, 3:211–216, 1961.

Hermann, J. S., The specific role of contact lenses in sensorimotor anomalies, *American Orthoptic Journal*, 16:30–43, 1966.

——— and B. S. Priestley, Bifoveal instability: the relationship to strabismic amblyopia, *American Journal of Ophthalmology*, 60(3):452–459, 1965.

Higgins, G. C., and K. F. Stultz, Frequency and amplitude of ocular tremor, *Journal of the Optical Society of America*, 43(12):1136–1140, 1953.

Hirsch, Monroe J., Functional amblyopia and social deprivation—a report on eight cases, *American Journal of Optometry and Archives of American Academy of Optometry,* 42(4):244–247, 1965.

Hoffstetter, H. W., Accomodative convergence in identical twins, *American Journal of Optometry and Archives of American Academy of Optometry,* 25(10):480–491, 1948.

Horwich, H., Anisometropic amblyopia, *American Orthoptic Journal,* 14:99–104, 1964.

Hubel, D. H., and T. N. Wiesel, Receptive fields of cells in striate cortex of very young, visually inexperienced kittens, *Journal of Neurophysiology,* 26(11):994–1002, 1963.

——— and ———, Binocular interaction in striate cortex of kittens reared with artificial squint, *Journal of Neurophysiology,* 28(11):1041–1059, 1965.

Hughes, William F. (ed.), *The Year Book of Ophthalmology, 1963–1964 Series.* Chicago, Year Book Medical Publishers, Inc., 1964.

Humphriss, D., Some notes on the treatment of amblyopia, *Dioptric Review,* XXXIX(4):313, 1937.

Hylkema, B. S., Flicker fusion frequency in a few eye disturbances, *Ophthalmologica,* 132(3):202–203, 1956.

Irvine, S. R., A simple test for binocular fixation, *American Journal of Ophthalmology,* 27(7):740–746, 1944.

———, Amblyopia ex anopsia; observations on retinal inhibition, scotoma, projection, light difference discrimination and visual acuity, *Transactions of the American Ophthalmological Society,* 46:527–575, 1948.

———, Measuring scotomas with the prism-displacement test in strabismus, retinal and neurologic conditions and glaucoma, *American Journal of Ophthalmology,* 61(5 Pt. II):1177–1187, 1966.

deJaeger, A., and J. Bernolet, Amblyopia ex anopsia treatment by pricking holes, *Ann. Oculi,* 189:734–735, 1956.

Jaffe, N. S., Some phenomena associated with amblyopia, *American Orthoptic Journal,* 14:123–130, 1964.

Jampolsky, A., B. C. Flom, F. W. Weymouth, and L. E. Moses, Unequal corrected visual acuity as related to anisometropia, *Archives of Ophthalmology,* 54(6):893–905, 1955.

Johnson, D. S. and J. Antuna, Atropine and miotics for treatment of amblyopia, *American Journal of Ophthalmology,* 60(5):889–891, 1965.

Jones, L. A., and G. C. Higgins, Some characteristics of the visual system of importance in the evaluation of graininess and granularity, *Journal of the Optical Society of America,* 37(4):217–263, 1947.

Jonkers, G. H., First impressions of treatment with the Euthyscope, *Ophthalmologica,* 132(5):322–326, 1956.

———, The examination of the visual acuity of children, *Ophthalmologica,* 136:140–144, 1958.

———, What is to be expected of amblyopia treatment? *Ophthalmologica,* 137(6):365–371, 1959.

Juler, F., Amblyopia from disuse, *Transactions of the Ophthalmological Society of the United Kingdom*, 41:129, 1921.

Kavner, R. S., Amblyopia evaluation and prognosis, *Optometric Weekly*, 57(28, 2nd section):7–13, 1966.

—— and I. B. Suchoff, *Pleoptics Handbook*. New York, Optometric Center of New York.

Keesey, Ülker T., Effects of involuntary eye movements on visual acuity, *Journal of the Optical Society of America*, 50(8):769–774, 1960.

Keiner, E. C. J. F., Pathogenesis of eccentric fixation, *American Journal of Ophthalmology*, 63(1):20–22, 1967.

Keiner, G. B. J., *New Viewpoints on the Origin of Squint*. The Hague, Martinus Nijhoff, 1951.

Kiff, R. D., and C. Lepard, Visual responses in premature infants, *Archives of Ophthalmology*, 75(5):631–633, 1966.

King, J. W., and L. D. Michael, Therapeutic orthoptics, *Journal of the American Optometric Association*, 36(4):335–343, 1965.

Kitao, J., Studies on the development of depth perception for near and distant objects in childhood, *Japanese Journal of Ophthalmology*, 4:67–76, 1960.

Koch, C. C., The Hall selection test as a diagnostic aid in amblyopic cases, *American Journal of Optometry and Archives of American Academy of Optometry*, 17(8):372–373, 1940.

Krajevitch, E., Des dangers de l'occlusion dans le traitement de l'amblyopie, *Bulletins et Mémoires de la Société française d'Ophtalmologie*, 62:249–255, 1962.

Kramer, M. E., *Clinical Orthoptics*, 2nd ed. St. Louis, Mo., C. V. Mosby Co., 1953.

Krill, A. E., Retinal function studies in hysterical amblyopia, *American Journal of Ophthalmology*, 63(2):230–237, 1967.

—— and F. W. Newell, The diagnosis of ocular conversion reaction involving visual function, *Archives of Ophthalmology*, 79(3):254–261, 1968.

Kunst, J. H., Red filter treatment of eccentric fixation, *Transactions of the Orthoptic Association of Australia*, pp. 61–62, 1963.

de Laet, H. A., and S. Szucs, Treatment of amblyopias with after-images, preliminary report, *Bulletin de la Société belge d'Ophtalmologie*, 112:227–236, 1956.

——, ——, and G. Leblois, Le traitement de la fixation extra-fovéale et de l'amblyopie par la méthode des post-images de Cüppers, *Bulletin de la Société belge d'Ophtalmologie*, 117:468–482, 1958.

Lancaster, W. B., Discussion of Lordan's paper, *Transactions of the Pacific Coast Oto-Ophthalmological Society*, 1940.

Landis, C., Something about flicker-fusion, *Scientific Monthly*, 73(5):308–314, 1951.

Lang, J., Über die Nach bildmethode von Cüppers bei der Behandlung der exzentrischen Fixation, *Ophthalmologica*, 131:261–262, 1956.

————, Amblyopia without strabismus and with inconspicuous small angle deviations, *Ophthalmologica*, 141:429–434, 1961.

Lawwill, T., The fixation pattern of the light-adapted and dark-adapted amblyopic eye, *American Journal of Ophthalmology*, 61(6):1416–1419, 1966.

————, Local adaptation in functional amblyopia, *American Journal of Ophthalmology*, 65(6):903–906, 1968.

————, and H. M. Burian, Luminance, contrast function and visual acuity in functional amblyopia, *American Journal of Ophthalmology*, 62(3):511–520, 1966.

Lazich, B. M., Amblyopia ex anopsia: a new concept of its mechanism and treatment, *Archives of Ophthalmology*, 39(2):183–193, 1948.

Leibowitz, H., The effect of pupil size on visual acuity for photometrically equated test fields at various levels of luminance, *Journal of the Optical Society of America*, 42(6):416–422, 1952.

Levinson, J. D., E. L. Gibbs, M. L. Stillerman, and M. A. Perlstein, Electroencephalogram and eye disorders, *Pediatrics*, 7(3):422–427, 1951.

————, and M. L. Stillerman, The correlation between electroencephalographic findings and eye disorders in children (abstract of paper presented at Central Association of Electroencephalographers, 1949), *Electroencephalography and Clinical Neurophysiology*, 2:226, 1950.

Linksz, Arthur, Pathophysiology of amblyopia, *Journal of Pediatric Ophthalmology*, 1(1):19–25, 1964.

———— and D. Guerry, III (eds.), *International Ophthalmology Clinics, Pleoptics; Light Coagulation*, Vol. 1, No. 4. Boston, Little, Brown & Co., 1961.

Lister, M. P., Amblyopia ex anopsia: approach and treatment, *American Orthoptic Journal*, 8:130–132, 1958.

Lowe, R. F., The use of atropine in the treatment of amblyopia ex anopsia, *Medical Journal of Australia*, 1:725–728, 1963.

Ludlam, W. M., Refractive interferences with management of normal binocular development, *Journal of the American Optometric Association*, 34(6):463–465, 1963.

Ludvigh, E., Effect of reduced contrast on visual acuity as measured with Snellen test letters, *Archives of Ophthalmology*, 25(3):469–474, 1941.

————, Visual mechanism in so-called amblyopia ex anopsia, *American Journal of Ophthalmology*, 25(2):213 ff., 1942.

————, Hypothesis concerning amblyopia ex anopsia (abstract of a paper presented before the New England Ophthalmological Society, Feb. 18, 1948), *Archives of Ophthalmology*, 42(2):397, 1950.

Lumbroso, B. D., and F. Proto, Le anomalie del senso cromatico nei soggetti ambliopici con fissazione eccentrica, *Bollettino d'Oculistica*, 42(11):699–718, 1963.

Lyle, T. Keith, and G. J. O. Bridgeman, *Worth and Chavasse's Squint*, 9th ed. London, Bailliere, Tindall, and Cox, 1959.

————, C. Douthwaite, and J. Wilkinson, *Abridged English Version of*

Sédan's Re-Educative Treatment of Suppression Amblyopia. Edinburgh and London, E. and S. Livingstone Ltd., 1960.

————, and S. Jackson, *Practical Orthoptics,* 4th ed. Philadelphia, Pa., Blakiston Co., 1953.

Mackensen, G., Das Fixationsverhalten amblyopischer Augen; elektroculographische Untersuchungen, *Albrecht von Graefe's Archiv für Ophthalmologie,* 159(2):200–211, 1957.

————, Blickbewegungen amblyopischer Augen: elektroculographische Untersuchungen, *Albrecht von Graefe's Archiv für Ophthalmologie,* 159(2):212–232, 1957.

————, Einfluss pleoptischer Behandlung auf die Blickbewegungen schwachsichtiger Augen, *Klinische Monatsblätter für Augenheilkunde,* 131(5):640–650, 1957.

————, Reaktionszeitmessungen bei Amblyopie, *Albrecht von Graefe's Archiv für Ophthalmologie,* 159(6):636–642, 1958.

————, Monoculare und binoculare statische Perimetrie zur Untersuchung der Hemmungsvorgänge beim Schielen, *Albrecht von Graefe's Archiv für Ophthalmologie,* 160(5):573–587, 1959.

————, Zur Phänomenologie und Pathogenese der exzentrischen Fixation: Antowort auf zwei Arbeiten von O. Oppel, *Albrecht von Graefe's Archiv für Ophthalmologie,* 166(1):87–100, 1963.

Maggi, C., Classification of amblyopia, *British Journal of Ophthalmology,* 43(6):345–360, 1959.

Malbràn, J. Tratamiento de la amblyopìa, *Archivos de Oftalmología de Buenos Aires,* 31(12):317–326, 1956.

Maraini, G., R. Franguelli, L. Pasino, and G. Diotti, The effect of total darkness on protein metabolism of the retina and the external geniculate body, *Bollettino d'Oculistica,* 42:175–182, 1963.

————, L. Pasino, and S. Peralta, Separation difficulty in amblyopia, *American Journal of Ophthalmology,* 56(6):922–925, 1963.

Marshall, R. L., and M. C. Flom, Amblyopia, visual acuity, and the Stiles-Crawford effect. Paper read before the annual meeting of the American Academy of Optometry, Los Angeles, Dec. 10, 1968.

Marx, E., and W. Trendelenburg, Über die Genauigkeit der Einstellung des Auges beim Fixieren, *Zeitschrift für Sinnesphysiologie,* 45:87–102, 1911.

Matteucci, P., Strabismic amblyopia, *British Journal of Ophthalmology,* 44(10):577–582, 1960.

————, G. Maraini, and S. Peralta, Modifications de la difficulté de séparation dand l'oeil amblyope strabique à luminance mésopique, *Archivos d'Ophtalmologie,* 23:655–658, 1963.

————, L. Pasino, and G. Maraini, Fixation in strabismus amblyopia, *Strabismus,* 2:71–113, 1964.

Maxwell, J. C., On the unequal sensibility of the foramen centrale to lights of different colours, *Report of the British Association for the Advancement of Science,* Pt. 2:12, 1856.

Mayweg, S., and H. H. Massie, Amblyopia ex anopsia (suppression amblyopia); a preliminary report of the more recent methods of treatment of amblyopia, especially when associated with eccentric fixation in cases of strabismus, British Journal of Ophthalmology, 42(5)257–269, 1958.

McCulloch, C., Discussion of Ramsay, Archives of Ophthalmology, 43(1):188, 1950.

McNeil, N. L., Patterns of visual defects in children, British Journal of Ophthalmology, 39(11):688–701, 1955.

Meyer, A. W., A report on six cases of juvenile functional amblyopia, Optometric Weekly, 57(41):33–34, 1966.

Miles, P. W., Flicker fusion frequency in amblyopia ex anopsia, American Journal of Ophthalmology, 32(6 Pt. II):225–230, 1949.

Miles, W. R., A functional analysis of regional differences in the human fovea, Science, 108:683, 1948.

———, On the central zone of the human fovea, Science, 109:441, 1949.

Miller, E. F., II, The nature and cause of impaired vision in the amblyopic eye of a squinter, American Journal of Optometry and Archives of American Academy of Optometry, 31(12):615–623, 1954.

———, Investigation of the nature and cause of impaired visual acuity in amblyopia, American Journal of Optometry and Archives of American Academy of Optometry, 32(1):10–28, 1955.

Miller, J. E., and L. Cibis, Clinical results with active amblyopia treatment, American Orthoptic Journal, 10:28–32, 1960.

———, L. C. Johnson, G. A. Ulett, and J. Hartstein, Photic driving in amblyopia ex anopsia, American Journal of Ophthalmology, 51(3):463–469, 1961.

Miller, R. G., Differential diagnosis of amblyopia with the modified ophthalmoscope, Journal of the American Optometric Association, 33(9):140–142, 1961.

Missotten, R., and J. Nelis, La fixation non fovéale du strabisme concomitant, Bulletin de la Société belge d'Ophtalmologie, 111:364–369, 1955.

Montague, R., and J. Walker, Contact lenses used as occluders, British Orthoptic Journal, 24:120–125, 1967.

Murroughs, T. R., Clinical Guide to Amblyopia Therapy. American Optometric Association, 1957.

———, and H. N. Walton, Differential diagnosis of amblyopia, Optometric Weekly, 43(14):535–539, 1952.

Nawratzki, I., E. Auerbach, and H. Rowe, Amblyopia ex anopsia: the electrical response in retina and occipital cortex following photic stimulation of normal and amblyopic eyes, American Journal of Ophthalmology, 61(3):430–435, 1966.

——— and A. Jampolsky, A regional hemiretinal difference in amblyopia, American Journal of Ophthalmology, 46(3 pt. I):339–344, 1958.

Naylor, E. J., and A. G. Wright, Incidence of amblyopia in children with strabismus, British Orthoptic Journal, 16:109–113, 1959.

von Noorden, G. K., Treatment of squint amblyopia with the after-image method, *American Journal of Ophthalmology*, 47(6):809–814, 1959.

————, Pathophysiology of amblyopia, Part II: diagnostic and therapeutic principles of pleoptics, *American Orthoptic Journal*, 10:7–16, 1960.

————, Reaction time in normal and amblyopic eyes, *Archives of Ophthalmology*, 66(5):695–701, 1961.

————, Bilateral eccentric fixation, *Archives of Ophthalmology*, 69(1):25–31, 1963.

————, Prophylaxis of amblyopia, *Journal of Pediatric Ophthalmology*, 1(4):35–38, 1964.

————, Sensory and motor factors in strabismic amblyopia, *American Orthoptic Journal*, 14:105–112, 1964.

————, Occlusion therapy in amblyopia with eccentric fixation, *Archives of Ophthalmology*, 73(6):776–781, 1965.

————, Pathogenesis of eccentric fixation, *American Journal of Ophthalmology*, 61(3):399–422, 1966.

————, Classification of amblyopia, *American Journal of Ophthalmology*, 63(2):238–244, 1967.

————, L. Allen, and H. M. Burian, A photographic method for the determination of the behavior of fixation, *American Journal of Ophthalmology*, 48(4):511–514, 1959.

————, and H. M. Burian, An electro-ophthalmolographic study of the behavior of the fixation of amblyopic eyes in light- and dark-adapted state; a preliminary report, *American Journal of Ophthalmology*, 46(1 Pt. II):68–77, 1958.

———— and ————, Visual acuity in normal and amblyopic patients under reduced illumination, *Archives of Ophthalmology*, I: Behavior of visual acuity with and without neutral density filter, 61(4):533–535, 1959; II: The visual acuity at various levels of illumination, 62(3):396–399, 1959.

———— and ————, Perceptual blanking in normal and amblyopic eyes, *Archives of Ophthalmology*, 64(6):817–822, 1960.

———— and M. B. Leffler, Visual acuity in strabismic amblyopia under monocular and binocular conditions, *Archives of Ophthalmology*, 76(2):172–177, 1966.

———— and R. M. C. Lipsius, Experiences with pleoptics in 58 patients with strabismic amblyopia, *American Journal of Ophthalmology*, 58(1):41–51, 1964.

———— and G. Mackensen, Pursuit movements of normal and amblyopic eyes: an electro-ophthalmographic study, *American Journal of Ophthalmology*, Part I: Physiology of pursuit movements, 53(2):325–336, 1962; Part II: Pursuit movements in amblyopic patients, 53(3):477–487, 1962.

————, and ————, Phenomenology of eccentric fixation, *American Journal of Ophthalmology*, 53(4):642–661, 1962.

————, and A. E. Maumenee, Clinical observations in stimulus-deprivation amblyopia (amblyopia ex anopsia), *American Journal of Ophthalmology*, 65(2):220–224, 1968.

Nordlöw, W., and S. Joachimsson, A screening test for visual acuity in four-year-old children, *Acta Ophthalmologica*, 40:453–462, 1962.

Nutt, A. B., Principles underlying the treatment of amblyopia, *British Orthoptic Journal*, 19:2–7, 1962.

Obal, A., Nutritional amblyopia, *American Journal of Ophthalmology*, 34(6):857–865, 1951.

Oppel, O., Über unsere gegenwärtigen Vorstellungen vom Wesen der funktionellen Schwachsichtigkeit, *Klinische Monatsblätter für Augenheilkunde*, 136(1):1–20, 1960.

————, Zur Phänomenologie der exzentrischen Fixation, *Klinische Monatsblätter für Augenheilkunde*, 141(3):161–169, 1962.

————, Stellungnahne zu der Veröffentlichung von G. Mackensen und G. K. von Noorden: "Zur Phänomenologie und Pathogenese der exzentrischen Fixation bei der Schielamblyopie," *Albrecht von Graefe's Archiv für Ophthalmologie*, 165(6):259–273, 1962.

————, Vergleichende Farbsinnuntersuchungenzwischen normalen und schielamblyopen Augen, *Albrecht von Graefe's Archiv für Ophthalmologie*, 165:387–391, 1963.

———— and D. Kranke, Vergleichende Untersuchunger über das Verhalten der Dunkeladaption normaler und schielamblyopen Augen, *Albrecht von Graefe's Archiv für Ophthalmologie*, 159(5):486–501, 1958.

Ordy, J. M., A. Latanick, T. Samorajski, and L. C. Massopust, Jr., Visual acuity in newborn primate infants, *Proceedings of the Society for Experimental Biology and Medicine*, 115:677–680, 1964.

Otwell, Harry C., *Therapeutic Orthoptics*. Fayetteville, Ark., 1958.

————, Conditioned tonotic treatment and macular generation, *Optical Journal and Review of Optometry*, XCVII(22):31–33; XCVII(23):27–28; XCVII(24):35–36, 1960; XCVIII(16):35–37, 1961.

————, The ribbon technique in cases of tropia, *Optical Journal and Review of Optometry*, C(21):21–22, 1963.

————, *Therapeutic Orthoptics: Conditioned Tonotic Treatment and Macular Generation*. Fayetteville, Ark., 1964.

————, Conditioned tonotic treatment and macular generation—a statistical view, *Optical Journal and Review of Optometry*, CI(8):33–40, 1964.

————, The "hidden threat" of amblyopia, *Optical Journal and Review of Optometry*, CII(20):41–44, 1965.

————, Therapeutic orthoptics, *Optometric World*, 53(9):28–32; 53(11):12–16, 1966.

Pajor, R., and Medgyaszay, Color sensitivity of strabismic-amblyopic eyes: a preliminary report, *Szemészet*, 101:41–43, 1964.

Parks, M. M., and D. S. Friendly, Treatment of eccentric fixation in children under four years of age, *American Journal of Ophthalmology*, 61(3):395–399, 1966.

Parsons-Smith, G., Activity of the cerebral cortex in amblyopia, *British Journal of Ophthalmology*, 37(6):359–364, 1953.

——, Flicker stimulation in amblyopia, *British Journal of Ophthalmology*, 37(7):424–431, 1953.

Pasino, L., On the factors leading to an eccentric type of fixation in strabismic amblyopia, *Ophthalmologica*, 143(6):431–437, 1962.

—— and G. Maraini, Le champ visuel central en vision monoculaire dans l'amblyopie, *Annales d'Oculistique*, 196(6):563–569, 1963.

—— and ——, Importance of natural test conditions in assessing the sensory state of the squinting subject, *British Journal of Ophthalmology*, 48(1):30–34, 1964.

——, ——, and M. Cordella, L'acuité visuelle dans l'amblyopie: I. Variations de l'acuité en fonction des tests employés, *Ophthalmologica*, 145(1):1–6, 1963.

Peckham, R. M., *Amblyopia*, Clinical Research Report No. 2, 4th ed. Detroit, Mich., Optometric Research Institute, 1941.

Perdriel, G., and F. Lods, L'électro-rétinographie dans l'amblyopie ex anopsia, *Annales d'Oculistique*, 196(5):485–496, 1963.

Perkins, E. S., Mechanism of amblyopia, *British Orthoptic Journal*, 15:16–22, 1958.

Phillips, C. I., Strabismus, anisometropia, and amblyopia, *British Journal of Ophthalmology*, 43(8)449–460, 1959.

Pistocchi, P., and O. Lamberti, Further statistical investigation on the relationship of refraction, ocular motility, and amblyopia, *Archives of Ottalmologia*, 66:253–258, 1962.

Polyak, Stephen, *The Retina*. Chicago, University of Chicago Press, 1941.

Potts, A. M., Retinotoxic and choroidotoxic substances, *Investigative Ophthalmology*, 1(3):290–303, 1962.

Priestley, B. S., Pleoptics at the New York Eye and Ear Infirmary, *American Orthoptic Journal*, 10:55–62, 1960.

——, H. M. Byron, and A. C. Weseley, Pleoptic methods in the management of amblyopia with eccentric fixation, *American Journal of Ophthalmology*, 48(4):490–502, 1959.

—— and J. S. Hermann, Visual acuity in dark-adapted patients, *Journal of Pediatric Ophthalmology*, 1(2):64–67, 1964.

——, ——, and M. Bloom, Amblyopia secondary to unilateral high myopia, *American Journal of Ophthalmology*, 56(6):926–932, 1963.

——, ——, and A. H. Nutter, Home pleoptics, *Archives of Ophthalmology*, 70(5):616–624, 1963.

Pritchard, R. M., Stabilized images on the retina, *Scientific American*, 204(6):72–78, 1961.

Pugh, M., Brightness perception and binocular adaptation, *British Journal of Ophthalmology*, 35(3):134–142, 1951.

——, Foveal vision in amblyopia, *British Journal of Ophthalmology*, 38(6):321–331, 1954.

——, Visual distortion in amblyopia, *British Journal of Ophthalmology*, 42(8):449–460, 1958.

——, Amblyopia and the retina, *British Journal of Ophthalmology*, 46(4):193–211, 1962.

Ramsay, R. M., Amblyopia ex anopsia, *Archives of Ophthalmology*, 43(1):188, 1950.

Randell, H. G., D. J. Brown and L. J. Sloan, Peripheral visual acuity, *Archives of Ophthalmology*, 75(4):500–504, 1966.

Rascati, E. J., and I. Suchoff, Pleoptics, the visuscope and eccentric fixation, *Journal of the American Optometric Association*, 32(1):39–45, 1961.

Rasch, E., H. Swift, A. H. Riesen, and K. L. Chow, Altered structure and composition of retinal cells in dark-reared mammals, *Experimental Cell Research*, 25:348–363, 1961.

Ratiu, E., and E. Reiter, Results obtained with the red filter method in the treatment of amblyopia with eccentric fixation, *Journal of Pediatric Ophthalmology*, 3(3):28–30, 1966.

Ratliff, F., The role of physiological nystagmus in monocular acuity, *Journal of Experimental Psychology*, 43:163–172, 1952.

—— and M. Fliegelman, Influence of fixation on the visual acuity, *Archives of Ophthalmology*, 12:475, 1934.

—— and L. A. Riggs, Involuntary motions of the eye during monocular fixation, *Journal of Experimental Psychology*, 40:687–701, 1950.

Reinecke, R. D., Objective and subjective testing of visual acuity in amblyopic patients, *American Orthoptic Journal*, 9:93–95, 1959.

—— and D. G. Cogan, Standardization of objective visual acuity measurements: Opticokinetic nystagmus vs. Snellen acuity, *Archives of Ophthalmology*, 60(3):418–421, 1958.

Riesen, A. H., Effects of stimulus deprivation on the development and atrophy of the visual sensory system, *American Journal of Orthopsychiatry*, 30(1):23–36, 1960.

Riggs, L. A., The measurement of normal ocular tremor by corneal reflection, *Journal of the Optical Society of America*, 42(4):287, 1952.

——, J. C. Armington, and F. Ratliff, Motions of the retinal image during fixation, *Journal of the Optical Society of America*, 44(4):315–321, 1954.

Ruben, M., A selective occluder, *British Orthoptic Journal*, 21:120–121, 1964.

Rubin, W. R., Reverse prisms in the treatment of strabismus and amblyopia, *American Orthoptic Journal*, 16:62–64, 1966.

Rucker, C. W., *The Interpretation of Visual Fields*, Home Study Course Manual, *American Academy of Ophthalmology and Otolaryngology*, 1954.

——, Tobacco amblyopia, *Proceedings of the Mayo Clinic*, 35(6):345–348, 1960.

Ruskell, G. L., Some aspects of vision in infants, *British Orthoptic Journal*, 24:25–32, 1967.

Saiduzzafar, H., and C. M. Ruben, Dark adaptation in amblyopes: a preliminary report, *British Orthoptic Journal*, 19:31–34, 1962.

—— and ——, Visual acuity thresholds in amblyopes, *British Journal of Ophthalmology*, 47(3):153–163, 1963.

Saraux, H., Anomalies of color perception as the cause of relative amblyopias of childhood, *Bulletin des Sociétés d'Ophtalmologie de France*, 76:115–121, 1963.

Sarrazin, L., First impressions of the treatment of amblyopia by Cüppers' method, *Bulletin des Sociétés d'Ophtalmologie de France*, 1:231–235, 1956.

Sauberli, R., Modern therapy of suppression amblyopia, *British Orthoptic Journal*, 19:8–12, 1962.

Schapero, M., Amblyopia ex anopsia, *American Journal of Optometry and Archives of American Academy of Optometry*, 38(9):509–530, 1961.

Schlossman, A., Pleoptics, *Eye, Ear, Nose and Throat Monthly*, 38(4):314–315, 1959.

—— and B. S. Priestley, Role of heredity in etiology and treatment of strabismus, *Archives of Ophthalmology*, 47(1):1–20, 1952.

Schmöger, E., and W. Müller, Das Elektroretinogramm und die corticale Uberleitungzeit bei Schielamblyopen, *Albrecht von Graefe's Archiv für Ophthalmologie*, 167:299–306, 1964.

Schwarting, B. H., Testing infants' vision, *American Journal of Ophthalmology*, 38(5):714–715, 1954.

Scully, J. P., Early intensive occlusion in strabismus with non-central fixation: Preliminary results, *British Medical Journal*, 2(12):1610–1612, 1961.

——, Non-central fixation in squinting children, *British Journal of Ophthalmology*, 45(11):741–753, 1961.

Sevrin, G., Treatment of amblyopia with after-images, *Bulletin de la Société belge d'Ophtalmologie*, 109:80–85, 1955.

——, Notions actuelles sur la physiopathologie et le traitement des amblyopies bilatérales, *Bulletin des Sociétés d'Ophtalmologie de France*, 1:21–39, 1956.

Sheridan, M. D., Diagnosis of visual defect in early childhood, *British Orthoptic Journal*, 20:29–36, 1963.

Sherman, M. E., and B. S. Priestley, The Haidinger brush phenomenon, a new clinical use, *American Journal of Ophthalmology*, 54(5):807–812, 1962.

Shipley, T., Haidinger's brushes in the clinical haploscope, *Archives of Ophthalmology*, 70(2):176–177, 1963.

Silvette, H., H. B. Haag, and P. S. Larson, Tobacco amblyopia, *American Journal of Ophthalmology*, 50(1):71–100, 1960.

Simon, K., Pleoptics, *Optometric Weekly*, 53(52):2515–2519, 1962.

Sjögren, H., A new series of tables for testing acuity in children, *Acta Ophthalmologica*, 17:67, 1939.

Slataper, F. J., Age norms of refraction and vision, *Archives of Ophthalmology*, 43(3):466–481, 1950.

Smith, G. G., H. B. Crasilneck, and C. W. Browning, A follow-up study of suppression amblyopia, *American Journal of Ophthalmology*, 52(5 Pt. I):690–693, 1961.

Smith, William S., *Clinical Orthoptic Procedure*. St. Louis, Mo., C. V. Mosby Co., 1950; 2nd ed., 1954.

————, Exanoptic and suppression amblyopia, *Archivos de la Sociedad Americana de Oftalmologia y Optometria*, 3(1):57–67, 1960.

————, The use of pleoptics in orthoptics, *American Journal of Optometry and Archives of American Academy of Optometry*, 38(1):28–39, 1961.

————, Pleoptics as an orthoptic procedure, *Journal of the American Optometric Association*, 33(12):355–358, 1961.

Sorsby, A., *Modern Ophthalmology*, Vol. 3. Washington, Butterworth and Co. Ltd., 1964.

Stanworth, A., Modified major amblyoscope, *British Journal of Ophthalmology*, 42(5):270–287, 1958.

———— and E. J. Naylor, Haidinger's brushes and the retinal receptors: with a note on the Stiles-Crawford effect, *British Journal of Ophthalmology*, 34(5):282–291, 1950.

Steer, J., Management of eccentric fixation: I. Children up to the age of 5 years, *British Orthoptic Journal*, 21:73–77, 1964.

Sternberg, A., and A. Bohar, A study on the occlusion therapy of eccentric fixation, *Ophthalmologica*, 141(3):229–235, 1961.

Straub, W., *Das Elektroretinogramm*. Stuttgart, Ferdinand Enke Verlag, 1961.

Stuart, J. A., and H. M. Burian, A study of separation difficulty: Its relationship to visual acuity in normal and amblyopic eyes, *American Journal of Ophthalmology*, 53(3):471–477, 1962.

Sugar, H. S., Suppression amblyopia, *American Journal of Ophthalmology*, 27(5): 469–476, 1944.

Sutcliffe, S., Prevention and treatment of amblyopia ex anopsia in the school health service, *British Orthoptic Journal*, 15:86–97, 1958.

Sutor, F. W., Suggestions for training amblyopia, *Optometric Weekly*, 50:1549–1551, 1959.

Swan, K. C., Esotropia following occlusion, *Archives of Ophthalmology*, 37(4):444–451, 1947.

————, Sensory physiology of binocular vision, *in Strabismus Ophthalmic Symposium* (I), edited by J. H. Allen. St. Louis, Mo., C. V. Mosby Co., 1950.

Swenson, A., Temporal occlusion in concomitant convergent strabismus, *American Orthoptic Journal*, 3:48–50, 1953; 8:45–47, 1958.

Szucs, S., Adaptometry in the amblyopia of strabismus, *Bulletin de la Société belge d'Ophtalmologie*, 116:287–298, 1957.

Talbot, S. A., and W. H. Marshall, Physiological studies in neural mechanisms of visual localization and discrimination, *American Journal of Ophthalmology,* 24(11):1255–1264, 1941.

Teräskeli, H., Untersuchungen über Amblyopie ohne Speigelbefund bei schielenden un nichschielenden Augen mittelst der Flimmermethode, *Acta Societatis Medicae Fennicae "Duodecim,"* Series B, 19(3):1 ff., 1934.

Theodore, F. H., R. M. Johnson, N. E. Miles, and W. H. Bonser, Causes of impaired vision in recently inducted soldiers, *Archives of Ophthalmology,* 31(5):399–402, 1944.

Thomas, Charles, and A. Bretagne, Considérations sur 70 cas d'amblyopie traités, apres echec d'autres procédés, par la méthode des post-images de Cüppers, *Bulletins et Mémoires de la Société française d'Ophtalmologie,* No. 5:521–525, 1956.

———— and A. Spielmann, À propos du test de Ammann, Burien, von Noorden, *Bulletin des Sociétés d'Ophtalmologie de France,* 63:544–549, 1963.

Tommila, V., Results in amblyopia treatment with Pleoptophor, *Acta Ophthalmologica,* 39(3):439–444, 1961.

Toselli, C., and G. Bertoncini, Analisi critica dei resultati a distanza consequiti in casi di ambliopia trattati con i metodi di Cüppers, *Annali di Ottalmologia e Clinica Oculistica* (Parma), 89(6):219–279, 1963.

von Tschermak-Seysenegg, *Introduction to Physiological Optics,* translation by P. Boeder. Springfield, Ill., Charles C Thomas, Publisher, 1952.

Tsutsui, J., Improvement of visual acuity by amobarbitol combined with pleoptics, *American Journal of Ophthalmology,* 62(6):1171–1176, 1966.

Urist, M. J., Eccentric fixation in amblyopia ex anopsia, *Archives of Ophthalmology,* 54(3):345–350, 1955.

————, Fixation anomalies in amblyopia ex anopsia, *American Journal of Ophthalmology,* 52(1):19–28, 1961.

VerLee, D. L., and I. Iacobucci, Pleoptics versus occlusion of the sound eye, *American Journal of Ophthalmology,* 63(2):244–250, 1967.

Victor, M., Tobacco-alcohol amblyopia: A critique of current concepts of this disorder, with special reference to the role of nutritional deficiency in its causation, *Archives of Ophthalmology,* 70(3):313–318, 1963.

———— and P. M. Dreyfus, Tobacco-alcohol amblyopia, *Archives of Ophthalmology,* 74(5):649–657, 1965.

————, E. L. Mancall, and P. M. Dreyfus, Deficiency amblyopia in the alcoholic patient, Archives of Ophthalmology, 64(1):1–33, 1960.

Viefhues, T. K., Prophylaxis and treatment of squint amblyopia in little children, *Klinische Monatsblätter für Augenheilkunde,* 131:827–829, 1957.

Wald, G., and H. M. Burian, The dissociation of form vision and light perception in strabismic amblyopia, *American Journal of Ophthalmology,* 27(9):950–963, 1944.

Walls, Gordon L., and R. W. Mathews, *New Means of Studying Color Blind-*

294 / Amblyopia

ness and Normal Foveal Color Vision. Berkeley and Los Angeles, University of California Press, 1952.

Walsh, F. B., *Clinical Neuro-Ophthalmology*, 2nd ed. Baltimore, Williams and Wilkins Co., 1957.

Walsh, T. J., Blindness in infants, *American Journal of Ophthalmology*, 62(3): 546–556, 1966.

Weekers, R., Critical frequency of fusion: clinical application, *in Modern Trends in Ophthalmology*, 3rd series, edited by Arnold Sorsby. New York, Paul B. Hoeber, Inc., 1955.

———, P. Moureau, J. Hacourt, and A. André, Contribution à l'étiologie du strabisme concomitant et de l'amblyopie par l'étude de jumeaux uni- et bivitellins, *Ophthalmologica*, 132(4):209–229, 1956.

Wekstein, L., Psychological aspects of amblyopia, *American Journal of Optometry and Archives of American Academy of Optometry*, 26(12): 511–518, 1949.

Wertheim, T. Über die indirekte Sehschärfe, *Zeitschrift für Psycholosie und Physiolosie der Sinnesorgan*, 7:172–189, 1894.

Wertheimer, M., Psychomotor coordination of auditory and visual space at birth, *Science*, 134:1692, 1961.

Westheimer, G., Visual acuity, *Annual Review of Psychology*, 16:359–380, 1965.

Weymouth, F. W., Visual sensory units and the minimal angle of resolution, *American Journal of Ophthalmology*, 46(1 Pt. II):102–113, 1958.

———, Visual acuity in children, *in Vision of Children*, edited by Monroe J. Hirsch and Ralph E. Wick. Philadelphia, Chilton Books, 1963, pp. 119–143.

———, D. C. Hines, L. H. Acres, J. E. Raaf, and M. C. Wheeler, Visual acuity within the area centralis and its relation to eye movements and fixation, *American Journal of Ophthalmology*, 11(12):947–960, 1928.

Wheeler, M. C., Strabismus amblyopia: Incidence and characteristics, *American Orthoptic Journal*, 6:13–18, 1956.

White, B. L., P. Castle, and R. Held, Observations on the development of visually directed reaching, *Child Development*, 35(2):349–364, 1964.

Wiesel, T. N., and D. H. Hubel, Effects of visual deprivation on morphology and physiology of cells in the cat's lateral geniculate body, *Journal of Neurophysiology*, 26(11):978–993, 1963.

——— and ———, Single-cell responses in striate cortex of kittens deprived of vision in one eye, *Journal of Neurophysiology*, 26(11):1003–1017, 1963.

——— and ———, Comparison of the effects of unilateral and bilateral eye closure on cortical unit responses in kittens, *Journal of Neurophysiology*, 28(11):1029–1040, 1965.

——— and ———, Extent of recovery from the effects of visual deprivation in kittens, *Journal of Neurophysiology*, 28(11):1060–1072, 1965.

Wild, B. W., Pleoptic techniques and visual training, *Journal of the American Optometric Association*, 32(6):457–460, 1961.

Wilson, G., and H. M. Katzin, Observations of pleoptic diagnosis and treatment, *American Orthoptic Journal*, 10:17–27, 1960.

———— and F. Walraven, Pleoptics and orthoptic analysis and treatment of fixation, *American Orthoptic Journal*, 12:97–108, 1962.

Wolff, Eugene, *The Anatomy of the Eye and Orbit*, 4th ed. New York, Blakiston Division, McGraw-Hill Book Co., Inc., 1955.

Wolin, L. R., and A. Dillman, Objective measurement of visual acuity using optokinetic nystagmus and electro-oculography, *Archives of Ophthalmology*, 71(6):822–826, 1964.

Woo, G., Incidence of amblyopia in grade school children in relation to age and sex. Paper read before the annual meeting of the American Academy of Optometry, Los Angeles, Dec. 10, 1968.

Worth, C., *Squint: Its Causes, Pathology, and Treatment*, 5th ed. Philadelphia, P. Blakiston's Son and Co., 1921.

Wybar, K., An introduction to the study of pleoptics, *British Orthoptic Journal*, 15:23–26, 1958.

Yasuna, E., Hysterical amblyopia in children, *American Journal of Diseases of Children*, 106:558, 1963.

Zanen, J., and S. Szucs, Les seuils achromatiques et chromatiques en vision centrale dans l'amblyopie strabique, *Bulletin de la Société belge d'Ophtalmologie*, 112 (Pt. 2):193–206, 1956.

Index

About the Author

Max Schapero, B.S., O.D., is Professor of Optometry and Lecturer in Orthoptics and Contact Lenses at the Los Angeles College of Optometry where he has also served as Director of the Contact Lens, Orthoptics, and Aniseikonia Clinics. He is a member of the American Academy of Optometry, a Diplomate in the Section on Contact Lenses, and has served as Chairman of the Section on Binocular Vision and Perception. He is currently Chairman of the Papers Program of the Contact Lens Section of the American Academy of Optometry, is a member of the Editorial Council of the *American Journal of Optometry and Archives of the American Academy of Optometry*, and is President of the California Chapter of the American Academy of Optometry. He is the author of numerous articles and original research papers in the fields of physiological optics, orthoptics, contact lenses, and aniseikonia, and is a co-editor of the first and second editions of the *Dictionary of Visual Science*.